Brittany & Jordan

In Micah's name,

Still hoping for change~

Eagle Feathers and Angel Wings:

Micah's Story

by

Shelley Muniz

Published in the United States by the Word Project Press of Sonora, CA

Requests for permission to make copies of any part of this work should be submitted online at info@wordprojectpress.com

Cover Design: Melody W. Baker

The Library of Congress has cataloged the Word Project edition as follows:
Muniz, Shelley.
Eagle Feathers and Angels Wings: Micah's Story / Muniz, Shelley —1st pbk ed.
2013934409

1. Health services accessibility--USA. 2. Medical care. 3. Health care reform--USA. 4. Leukemia in children. 5. Children--death. 6. Mothers and sons--USA. 7. Bereavement. 8. Loss (Psychology). 9. Grief. RA393.M86 2012

ISBN-13: 978-0989068208
ISBN-10: 0989068208

* The events and issues in *Eagle Feathers and Angel Wings: Micah's Story* are real, but in some instances the author has changed the names of individuals and places.

"In the battle against their son Micah's leukemia, the Chase family faced an unexpected foe in addition to the disease itself: their insurer's refusal to pay for the bone marrow transplant that offered Micah his best chance at recovery. *Eagle Feathers and Angel Wings: Micah's Story* is a loving tribute to a life cut tragically short, but its revelations about the difficulties ordinary Americans face in accessing critical medical treatments are deeply unsettling. I hope we can learn from Micah the dire necessity of overhauling the health care system to ensure no other child is denied the opportunity to grow up healthy and strong."

--President Bill Clinton
May 2008

"Parents, professionals, politicians of all stripes, and college students -- should read this book. Anyone claiming to be a responsible adult, citizen, parent, or professional should make it an imperative read. Although the story *is* an undeniable tragedy, the book should not be read as an exercise in entering the world of a family's private sorrow. The book should be read as a case study in adult-citizen-parental whistle blowing.

Our institutions are unlikely to self-correct in the absence of a demand to do so. Micah's story--and others like it--should mobilize such a demand. It should arouse anger and outrage, a strong commitment to understand more than we do about how society works, and a willingness to question and abandon if necessary all kinds of parochial prejudices. These should bring about something like the development of a nationwide whistleblower clearinghouse to serve as a database for collecting toxic institutional practices, so that these can be documented without people fearing retaliation. Perhaps most important, there needs to be consequences, especially for institutions and the professions, for silence and/or the manufacture of misleading institutional representation."

--Paula K. Clarke, Ph.D.
American Anthropological Association
Oxford University Press Award
Anthropology, 2008

"Eagle Feathers and Angel Wings chronicles the gradual descent of a happy family into an abysm of illness. The story itself is compelling, but Muniz's beautiful use of language, her vulnerability in expressing emotion, and her hard-earned insights make this a must-read. Here is an author unafraid to express her truth with a poet's tongue, written in heart's blood."

--Suzan Still,
Author of *Commune of Women* and *Fiesta of Smoke*

"This compelling story of a young boy's tragic battle with cancer provides an intimate view of the ways in which our health insurance system forsakes children and their families. While facing urgent medical needs, Micah's family faces heavy medical costs, struggles to comprehend and respond to decisions by the health insurance system, and consequent delays in treatment."

--Laura Lein, Ph.D.
School of Social Work
Department of Anthropology
The University of Texas at Austin

This book is dedicated to
my sons, Micah and Nick

--And to all children living with cancer,
their parents and siblings--

"As a kid I fell hard into illness
At fourteen, I have to stand as a man."

--Micah Chase, 1993

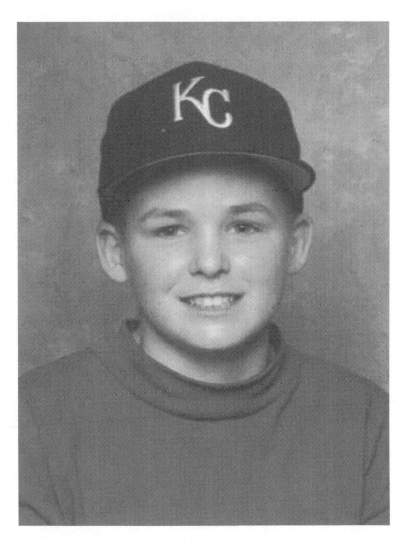

Micah Chase, November 1991

Chapter 1

It was June of 1991, summer vacation. We were playing a family game of Monopoly. Del was playfully cheating, the kids were laughing; I had declared mom's rules by default (Mom gets a free get-out-of-jail pass, just 'cause). Dinner was still settling in our stomachs -- individual pizzas made with English muffins, sauce, pepperoni, cheeses, and olives. The green salad on the side was a given, as I had been coaxed into an entrée of questionable nutritional value. Whooping with delight, Micah had just declared himself the owner of both Boardwalk and Park Place when the phone rang.

"Shelley," Dr. George said, "we've received the results of Micah's blood tests. You need to take him to Children's Hospital in Oakland. They want to see him right away."

"What?"

"You need to drive Micah to Oakland to the Children's Hospital," Dr. George repeated.

"Why?" I asked hesitantly. "Are you sure?"

"There was a problem with Micah's blood tests, and yes, I'm sure."

I turned away from my husband and children, trying to hide my concern. "Okay. Well…We'll go in the morning, first thing?" I twisted the phone cord around my arm, once, twice. Micah was winning at Monopoly; we had rented a video, *Kindergarten Cop*, to watch later.

"No, Shelley. Tonight. They want to see him tonight. And Shelley?" Dr. George's voice sounded grim; it was a tone I had never heard from the pediatrician who had taken care of my children since their births. "Drive carefully," he said. "If there were an accident, if Micah got hurt…his blood counts are so low…Shelley…he could bleed to death."

Micah was twelve, Nick, ten, Del and me, side-stepping through our forties with ease. We had a nice home, seven acres of land where the kids romped and played. Micah and Nick were mountain boys, raised on the top of Big Hill, a single hill named for what it was, standing tall and picturesque behind the town of Sonora, California. We worked hard for our property, built our home ourselves, each board and nail pounded by Del and me, sisters, brother-in-laws, and parents. Micah and Nick hefted their little hammers as well, nailing in floorboards, wall braces and deck railings as they could manage.

Our land was their paradise. They had tree forts and hideouts under the Manzanita bushes. Their Tonka trucks and most of my Tupperware containers were scattered near rocks and under shrubs, anywhere they might find bugs, frogs, lizards, anything that crawled, hissed, or looked like an adventure. We had two dogs, three cats, three goats, various chickens and ducks, an Iguana named Iggy, a donkey on occasion, a horse on loan from my sister Jan. I had a huge vegetable garden and fruit trees: apple, nectarine, peach, plum, and pomegranate. There was a swing set Del made out of logs; it was large and sturdy. A trampoline.

Rope swings galore. We camped, we swam. The kids played sports at school. I cooked well-balanced meals. I read books to both children every day, had night-time rituals filled with stories, songs, and lots of snuggles.

Del and I were good parents. We had great kids. Both of them were healthy from the day they were born, suffering little more than a head cold, the stomach flu. I took them in for yearly physicals and dental exams. They rarely missed a day of school, had even earned perfect attendance awards through most of their elementary school years.

Perfect kids. Perfect teeth. Perfect bodies.

And then I got the phone call from Dr. George.

"This could be something simple, right? I mean, this isn't..." I stopped myself mid-sentence, watching Micah's eyes.

"Try not to worry," Dr. George said. "Just get him to the hospital, and we'll go from there."

Don't worry. Yeah, right.

I had taken Micah to the pediatrician multiple times that year for leg cramps, lack of energy, unexplained headaches. Normally, this was a kid who traveled through life at full throttle. Midway through the 6th grade, he was running at half-steam. During wrestling matches at school, he would kind of stall out -- gritting his teeth, body arched, leg muscles stretched tight, he would get his opponent near to a pin, have the boy's shoulders close to the mat, but could not make that final push to get him down. While hiking, rather than run ahead, he fell behind. Playing baseball, in his position at first-base, I would see him lean down and rub his legs, miss a ball he normally would have caught. Micah was usually the first one up in the morning, dressed and ready for school, smiling, with his backpack filled and propped by the front door. He was spunky, always happy and full of fun. In his last weeks of 6th grade, he became moody, complaining about little things, had difficulty concentrating on his homework, and was easily distracted from his usual routine. He stayed in bed until I woke him by kissing his cheek, reminding him that it was a school day.

And there were the bruises.

I had noticed them on the sides of his knees, his elbows. "Something is wrong," I told Dr. George. "This isn't normal. These bruises are huge."

"Shelley, calm down. He's an active twelve-year-old. That's all. Relax. Sit back and enjoy the ride through his adolescence."

That spring we picnicked at Pinecrest and hiked around the lake. We had cousins up to play. Nick laughed at Micah, wearing his new 'shades' and M.C. Hammer pants, listening to Eddie Van Halen while he rode his bike over some jumps they had rigged up on a hillside out by the garage. We went to San Francisco with friends, drove down Lombard Street, the 'Crookedest Street in the World', rode cable cars from the Wharf to Market Street and back, went to Pier 39 for lunch. Micah kept up with Jenny, Tommy, and Nick, but his stride was off, his skin looked pale. "Look at his face, compared to Jenny's," I told my friend Terry. "Something's not right."

"What do the doctors say?" Terry asked.

"They say nothing's wrong."

"Shelley, you know Micah better than anyone. If you feel like something is wrong, listen to your instincts. Insist that they do something different, another kind of test, maybe."

When school let out for the summer, Micah didn't want to attend the end-of-the-year party. I urged him to go, and he finally relented, but once we were there he barely left my side. "I just want to be with Nick today," he said, transforming Dinobots with his brother while his friends swam and played volleyball. "Mama," he said later, as we were packing up to go, "I don't know what's wrong. I feel like I'm dying inside."

My heart beat faster. My skin rippled with goose bumps head to toe.

I phoned the doctor as soon as we got home, insisting on more tests. Dr. George had us go to the hospital and get some lab work done, blood draws, a urinalysis. I had nearly forgotten that we were waiting for the results when the call came.

Go. Go now. Don't wait. Shelley -- if you get in an accident, Micah could bleed to death.

While Del talked with Dr. George, I packed a suitcase full of things, silly things, anything; Micah's things. I made arrangements with my sister to come over and watch Nick. The two of them stood on the porch, waving goodbye, biting lips, eyes blank and fearful, as Del and I drove off in the dark with Micah belted securely in the backseat of our car.

Chapter 2

Children's Hospital. It was a foreign land right from the start. Getting across the border required coming up with answers to a battery of unending questions. A pop quiz. I should have known all that stuff, but I couldn't think clearly enough to remember my own name.

Yes, Micah had had all his shots. No, I could think of nothing he had been exposed to within the last six weeks. My head was spinning. I didn't understand what the admission's clerk was asking. The tag on her jacket read Madge. The name, along with a strong southern accent, triggered something comically compulsive within the depths of my despair. Lips pursed, I babbled to myself: *Yes, Madge, he's extremely active, and he's always been so healthy; he's a smart kid, he wouldn't do anything crazy, honest Madge, this is my son Micah we're talking about. He has a good head on his shoulders.*

I searched the woman's eyes. What I wanted was for Madge to check things over and say, "Oh, I'm sorry, Mrs. Chase, there's been a mistake. Your son is as healthy as a horse. Go home and enjoy the rest of your life."

When Madge asked for our insurance information, I relaxed a little. The card I held in my hand was something I could present to her with certainty. "I've had this policy for ten years through my work," I said, as she noted the company, the type of plan, took photocopies of my personal and group ID numbers. "Oakland Children's Hospital is listed as a PPO provider, so I don't anticipate you'll have any problems," I added, feeling secure in that statement at least.

Madge handed me a plastic blue card. Micah's card. It had his name on it. "Don't lose it," she warned. "This is the lifeline for communication around here. They stamp it just like they would a credit card."

"Oh, great," I said, feeling uneasy again.

"We have a bed ready for him in Oncology."

What was Oncology, anyway? I tried to shake the attitude. It was not Madge's fault, but it was so difficult. My mind was waging an emotional battle; I felt lightheaded and close to tears.

"Take the main elevator from the lobby to the fifth floor, and then follow the arrows from the elevator toward the nurses' station," Madge said. "Someone will show you where to go from there."

"Thank you," I squeaked out, my voice small, mousy.

People were milling about everywhere. Wheelchairs carrying children in different phases of treatment rolled past us, pushed by parents with all-knowing eyes. I saw their stares and felt their looks of pity -- a new member of the club. I tried not to look at them, to acknowledge them in any way because to do so would be to admit that I, that Micah, was in the same boat as they were. It was more than I could handle.

The smell of disinfectant met us as we got off the elevator and walked onto the main corridor of the fifth floor. A nurse, blue chart in hand, was there to greet us as

7

promised. "You must be Micah," she said, smiling. "My name is Debbie. And yours?" she asked, turning to me and Del.

"I'm Shelley Chase. And this is my husband, Del. We're Micah's mom and dad."

"Hello," Del said.

"So nice to meet you," Debbie said, offering her hand to each of us. "Now, if you'll follow me, I'll get Micah settled."

The room was spacious with its own private bathroom, a single bed, small bureau, scrub sink, and window seat beneath a large window that looked out over the rooftops of neighboring buildings. Debbie pulled back the covers on the bed, laid out a hospital gown and slippers, and then went to the sink to wash her hands. "You'll be meeting lots of folks, Micah," she explained. "Doctors, nurses, interns -- people will be coming and going all the time. Sounds icky, I know, but actually it's better for you in the long run -- a lot more brain power working on trying to get you well. Okay so far?"

"I guess. The brain power part, that's cool." Turning to me with a sly smile, Micah pushed the button control that moved the bed up and down, back and forth, intending to play with his newly discovered toy whether I gave my permission or not.

Debbie laughed. "Oh, you're gonna be a feisty one. That's good. I like that -- the feistier the better."

I became watchful of the expression on Micah's face. His eyes were focused, his smile, steady and sincere. As Debbie talked, he was clearly intent on understanding her explanations, each description she gave of the events that

8

would follow. I struggled to catch up, having missed parts of the conversation due to my mindfulness of Micah.

"You'll be getting lots of tests," Debbie continued, uninterrupted. "What that means is lots of blood work, lots of pokes. Is that okay with you?"

"Not really," Micah said, smiling. "Be gentle," he teased. "I bruise easily."

Debbie laughed, and then turned to me and Del. "We're going to draw some blood, so we can see how things look now compared with the lab results you had done in Sonora this afternoon."

I nodded my head, closed my mouth and pinched my nose; I blew to stabilize the pressure in my ears, hoping it would make a difference in what I heard.

"As you know, Micah's platelets are very low. He'll need a transfusion, but the doctor will talk with you more about that later."

"Transfusion?" Micah sat up a little straighter, staring directly at Debbie. "I'm going to need a blood transfusion?"

"Yes," Debbie said. "We want to get you feeling better, okay?"

"Why do I need a transfusion?" Debbie looked surprised, but I was not. My son; it was his nature to question everything.

"Well," she said, "your blood doesn't have enough platelets. That's why you've been bruising so easily."

"So, you're going to give me some blood? Whose blood?"

Debbie laughed again. "Yes," she said, "we're going to give you some blood, and it will come from a local donor."

"How exactly, does that work?"

9

"We'll insert an IV in your arm, and you'll get the blood through the IV."

"Can I be his donor?" I asked.

"We'd like to ask you to wait on that. As Micah's parents, your blood may be needed later on, for a multitude of reasons. So for now, we'll use blood from our donor bank, all right?" She turned to Del. "The window seat doubles as a bed. Normally, we only allow one parent to sleep in the room, but I'll make special arrangements so you can both stay, at least temporarily. You may have to camp on the floor," she explained.

Del shrugged his shoulders and glanced at me. "Fine," he told her. "We can make it work, no problem."

Two doctors wearing long white coats came into the room. Micah sat cross-legged on the bed. They introduced themselves to him first, and then to Del and me.

Dr. James Feusner was a tall, slender man, formal in speech and serious in stature. His manner affirmed his position as the head of Pediatric Oncology. Dr. Machela Irwin was his assistant.

I felt myself shrinking. My heart was pounding, my throat constricting to the point no words would come out of my mouth. The only acknowledgement I could give both doctors at that moment was a nod.

Dr. Feusner led off with a round of questions while Dr. Irwin took notes. He started with the simple things, speaking directly to Micah. "How old are you? How tall? Do you know how much you weigh, Micah?" I watched Dr. Feusner perform a visual exam while he verbally probed for answers. "What are your hobbies? Where do you play after school? Any areas near the house that could be considered unsafe, anything you could have ventured into?"

Dr. Feusner lifted Micah's arm to check the bruises.

"Was there anything abnormal about your pregnancy?" Dr. Feusner asked me. "How was your health before your pregnancy with Micah and after?"

"I had easy pregnancies with both my kids. I didn't even have morning sickness, nothing like that at all. I've always been healthy. The kids, Del and I, get colds, the flu once in awhile, but that's it."

Dr. Feusner nodded, taking mental notes. "Tell me about any illnesses you had as a child. Did your mother take any medication during her pregnancy with you?"

"I had the chickenpox and the measles when I was little. My mother never mentioned anything about taking medication while she was pregnant. I'll check with her though."

"How's your health, Del? Did you have any illnesses that you know of as a child?"

"Chickenpox, and measles, tonsillitis, but nothing else, I'm sure."

The questions continued, but there were no firm conclusions to draw.

Normal pregnancy. Normal kid. Normal. Normal. Normal.

"Micah, as I'm sure Debbie told you, we're going to start with some blood tests. That okay with you?" Dr. Feusner asked.

Micah nodded his head, listening intently, having heard the word 'pokes' more than once. He grimaced, preparing himself. "My body, my decision?" he asked me.

I nodded, yes.

11

"Okay," he said. "Let's do it."

So like Micah, I thought again, always alert and in charge of his world. I could envision him as a one-year-old, cocking his head to the side, assessing sounds, sights, smells. He always tongue-tasted his food before putting it in his mouth and decided ahead of time whether to give it his full attention. Eyes intent, quivering with anticipation, he touched everything within reach. Our dog had a litter of puppies, and I couldn't keep Micah out of her box. Every time I turned around he was sitting with those puppies, running his hand over their soft coats, loving, snuggling, kissing their little heads. From the moment he could talk, he questioned everything. "What's dis? Dis?" he asked, pointing to his Sippy cup, and then his highchair, the couch, the front door, a tree, a flower, a dragonfly, a bird. Once he realized there were names for the things he loved, he couldn't get enough; he would toddle around the house and outside in the yard, pointing, calling on me with urgency to provide words that fit the sights, shapes, and textures around him.

Micah looked at me from his hospital bed with his hungry, precocious eyes, wanting answers, hoping for the peace of mind I had always been able to provide. As a mother, I felt empty and broken; I had no insight, no Band-Aid to offer as a placebo, nothing tangible I could give him but my smile and a kiss on the cheek.

Dr. Feusner smiled for the first time since he walked into the room. "I like a kid who takes charge," he said. "It's not often I see that in here."

"I want to be a doctor, maybe of sports medicine," Micah said.

12

"That's wonderful," Dr. Feusner said. "Let's get you fixed up, so you can do just that."

I smiled again, liking his answer. My heart felt a little lighter because of it.

Del was fidgeting nervously beside Micah's bed. He looked at the IV pump, turning it side to side on its rolling pole, inspecting with his mechanic's eye to get a grasp of how it worked. He gripped the foot railing of Micah's bed, shaking it slightly. "What do you think, Dr. Feusner?" he asked.

"We don't know. What we do know is that Micah's blood counts are very low. We're going to need to give him platelets as soon as possible. We won't transfuse with red blood until tomorrow afternoon."

A murky haze filled my eyes, distorting my vision. The room was spinning. Platelets. Transfusions. Red blood. Panic. It suddenly felt like they were feeding us information a piece at a time. Debbie had mentioned a platelet transfusion but said nothing about red blood cells.

"What we also know," Dr. Feusner said, "is that Micah has none of the classic symptoms that goes along with some of the childhood diseases we would normally look for under these circumstances. No swollen glands, no fever, or nausea."

"Yes, that's what our family doctor said."

"He was right," Dr. Feusner confirmed. "We'll need to do some more conclusive testing, of course but first, the blood draw, and then we need to raise his platelet count. If you will just sign these consent forms for the transfusions, we'll get things moving."

Sign on the dotted line. I could barely read the writing

on the paper he had handed me, let alone scratch my signature on the dotted line. I hesitated before signing, searching Dr. Feusner's eyes for hidden messages.

Debbie came back with a lab technician to draw the blood. Micah flinched slightly as she filled tube after tube. We began the waiting game. Every process took forever. The nursing staff was very thoughtful under the circumstances, bringing in extra towels, juice for Micah, in and out, in and out, all this going on while Debbie inserted an IV into Micah's arm, readying him for the transfusion that would follow. Hours passed before we got word from the blood bank; they had called in a special donor, one who often gave blood for the children at the hospital. The platelets would not be ready until early the next morning.

At half past midnight, Micah was finally allowed to sleep. I lay down in the window seat as Del left the room in search of coffee and in desperate need of exercise after hours of sitting in one position. In the white silence that followed his exit, I took a deep breath of hospital air.

Nothing to it. Stale. Antiseptic. Suffocating. Tears poured -- and prayers -- every prayer I could think of: Help me! Help my child. Please.

Chapter 3

Morning came none too soon. After a sleepless night, the nurse's station was gearing up for a shift change. People were on the move; I could see them through the window facing the corridor, checking charts, exchanging information. Maybe with the changing of the guard we would get some answers.

Someone knocked softly on the door. Micah turned over and sat up, forgetting for a moment about the tube connected to his hand. "Ouch!"

"Good morning, Buddy," Del said, as he entered the room.

Micah grinned. "Dad?" Where have you been?"

"Just cruisin' the halls. You know me. Can't sit still." Del handed me a large glass of orange juice and gave another one to Micah.

"Thanks," Micah said and took a big drink. "My breakfast comes special delivery," he added between gulps. "I even got to pick what I wanted, scrambled eggs or French toast."

"I hope you picked French toast. I've been casing this joint, and the word is, the eggs are hospital issue and about as gross as you can get." Del grinned.

"I ordered the French toast."

15

"Lucky dog."

There was another knock, this one more purposeful. Dr. Feusner entered the room with Micah's chart tucked under one arm. "How are you feeling, young man?"

"All right."

"Good. Glad to hear it."

"What's next?" Del asked.

"That's what I came to talk with you about," Dr. Feusner explained. "More blood tests for now. We'll also give Micah his transfusions, and over the next couple of days, monitor his blood counts and evaluate the results. Later, we'll take a look at his bone marrow."

Del raised his eyebrows, questioningly.

"To look at Micah's bone marrow -- what does that involve?" I asked.

"What that means is, when his platelet level is up, and we're ready to go, I'll extract some fluid from inside his hip bone using a needle designed especially for that purpose." He turned to Micah. "Before the procedure, Debbie will give you some medication that will make you feel very sleepy. She'll also give you some pain medication to keep you as comfortable as possible."

Micah frowned.

"Don't worry," Dr. Feusner told him. "I've done a lot of bone marrow aspirates, and I've been told I'm pretty good at it." He smiled and patted Micah's leg.

"Now, let's get those platelets aboard so you'll feel a little better, okay? You talk to Debbie for a bit, Micah. I need your mom and dad to come with me to look over and sign some paperwork."

Dr. Feusner led Del and me to a small conference room

16

with a long table strewn with papers. He motioned for us to sit. "I need you to know, Mrs. Chase, Mr. Chase, we still have no idea what we're looking at here."

"Why will you be testing Micah's bone marrow?" The words stuck together as they came out of my mouth.

"So far, we don't have much to go on. Everything we've checked for has tested out negative. Hopefully," Dr. Feusner continued, "looking at his marrow will give us the answers we need." He handed me a consent form for a bone marrow aspirate.

I scanned the first paragraph. 'Children's Hospital. Oncology Unit, 5th floor. Children's Cancer Ward.' I breathed deeply and swallowed my fear. It was just a consent form, nothing more. Just another piece of paper that made no sense. I signed blindly in my hurry to get back to Micah.

The hall was long and wide with doors lining both sides of the corridor. Children in wheelchairs and attached to IV poles sat outside their rooms, getting a respite from their beds while nurses changed sheets and blankets and replenished closets with supplies: clean towels, fresh nightgowns, alcohol pads, sterile drapes, gauze, and tape. A young boy, maybe four or five years old, bent and bandaged, raised his hand as we walked by, saying hello without speaking, smiling broadly as I waved back.

When we reached Micah's room, he was in a wheelchair as well. Debbie was administering his platelets. The transfusion went faster than I thought it would. Twenty minutes later, Micah was unhooked from the tubing connecting him to the empty platelet bag and was ready to sleep. Del went out into the hallway and to the pay phone to call his parents, his co-workers at the Tuolumne County Road Department. When he was finished, I took my turn, phoning the superintendent at Belleview School to explain that Micah might not be there for the start of classes and that I might not be there to start my fall assignment as kindergarten aide and school librarian.

Then I phoned my mother. "Tell Micah, this is a heck of a way to get attention," Grandma Nellie teased, trying to lighten my spirit, to ease my mind. "Tell him I love him," she added, tearfully. "And that I'll see him soon."

For the next two days, Micah had tests and more tests: blood draws, a chest x-ray, urinalysis, endless lab work. Our proof of insurance, the blue *credit card* we were given when Micah was admitted to the hospital was stamped or swiped and documented for hospital billing so often I placed it in a bureau drawer beside his bed for easy access.

Nick, Grandma Nellie, and my sisters, Jan and Carol arrived for a visit mid-morning of the third day just as Micah was wheeled back into his room after the bone marrow aspirate performed by Dr. Feusner.

"*Pieze* a cake. Didn't feel a thing," Micah told Nick, speech slurred, eyelids heavy from the anesthesia.

I stepped forward, reaching out and then back, not knowing whether to help or stand aside as the technician settled Micah into bed. I rubbed my temples, trying to dull the ache in my head, finally settling in a chair at Micah's bedside. Nick sat on my lap, clicking his tongue, humming a little nonsense song. I pulled him closer, nuzzling my face in his soft brown hair. The familiar scent of Johnson's Baby Shampoo calmed my nerves. No tears, I reminded myself.

18

No tears.

Micah hummed along with Nick and laughed, mumbling something about cheeseburgers and French fries. His eyes fluttered and then closed as I adjusted the blanket under his chin. Nick stopped humming and laid his head against my chest. We stayed that way, quiet and contemplative, until Dr. Feusner arrived with the test results. "The bone marrow aspirate was inconclusive," he reported, speaking softly while Micah slept.

"That's good, isn't it?" I asked.

"Yes," he said, "but we need to look further. We need to test Micah for different types of anemia, including Paroxysmal nocturnal hemoglobinuria -- hemolysis -- a breakdown of red blood cells that happens at night."

"Oh," I said. "Hemolysis," I repeated. I knew nothing of anemia, but the word slid over my tongue, sounded less threatening than other prognoses. I latched on to the disease and made it Micah's. "That has to be it," I said hopefully. "We'll be home in no time," I promised Nick.

The first week passed, and a multitude of doctors drifted through Micah's room, all asking the same questions, each of them wanting to hear firsthand the story of our lives. The results of the anemia testing, the test for hemolysis came back negative, and I grew more anxious, less cautious with my concerns. I questioned Debbie. "Have you heard anything? Do you have any idea what could be happening? He'll be okay, won't he? I mean, this isn't anything too serious, is it?"

The nursing staff remained supportive, but our patience wore thin, all but Micah's that is; his ability to endure never faltered. He cracked jokes and kept a positive attitude, listening intently as the doctors spoke to him, wanting to understand everything that had anything to do with his health. Good friends traveled the distance from Sonora to Oakland; we received an avalanche of calls and get-well cards. One wall of Micah's hospital room was covered by a giant green poster filled with good wishes, painted and signed by his classmates, bordered by pictures and notes from Nick, cousins Kip, Katy, Levi, and Season, and photos of the kids' dog, Butchy.

After twelve days with no diagnosis, Dr. Feusner suggested it was time to do another bone marrow aspirate. Carol, Katy, and Grandma Nellie came an hour before the procedure was scheduled to begin, armed with a goody basket full of games and magazines. Micah's eyes lit up. It was the perfect diversion. "How's Kip?" he asked Carol as he dug through the basket, checking things out, smiling.

"Good," Carol told him. "He misses you, though. He's ready to go find someone with chickenpox, get himself sick, get it over and done with -- so he can come visit you!" Carol chuckled, and so did Micah. Katy had had the chickenpox, but Kip hadn't; if he was exposed to the disease unknowingly, if there was a single blister anywhere, one sneeze, one touch, one exhaled breath, there would be serious problems on the fifth floor. Chicken pox was bad news for children with compromised immune systems. It could be deadly. Our decision to keep Kip at home had been difficult for both Micah and Kip, but it was necessary.

As we talked, a lab technician searched dutifully for a fresh spot from which he could find a vein strong enough to deliver Micah's intravenous anesthetic medication. His choices were limited; Micah's arms resembled pincushions; black and blue, dotted with reddish-purple petechiae, each one a testimony to a different needle.

I sat silently by as a solitary tear rolled down Micah's cheek. It was the first indication I'd had that he was feeling any discomfort. I stroked his hair and kissed his forehead, noting his concern, trying to reassure him as best I could. Looking into Micah's eyes was like looking into my own; they changed color with the light, sometimes green with a tinge of blue, sometimes more hazel though, like Del's. His lips were my lips, full and rosy. His hair was my hair, down to the perfectly swirled cowlick near the crown of his head, his soft brown waves.

The night shift came on board just as the drug took hold. Nurse Tom, Debbie's relief person, whispered and laughed as he wheeled Micah down the hall. Tom's sense of humor matched Micah's joke for joke and was a distraction from the mundane, a sideshow that kept Micah's mind off the reality of his situation. Watching Tom was like watching a whirlwind move through the place, rearranging, reorganizing, checking to make sure everything was being done to his satisfaction.

After less than an hour, Tom returned to announce that the procedure had gone well and was over. "The kid's done his part. Never let out a whimper. Even drugged up, the fact is he never stopped talking." Tom laughed. "Had Doc Feusner chuckling, and that's unheard of around here."

Tom's comments about Micah's sense of humor were appreciated, but no one in the room felt like laughing. I pictured Micah dressed as a mummy for Halloween one year, a Christmas elf in a parade down the main street in

21

Sonora: I could see him making faces through the picture window in our living room at home, wagging his bottom, wiggling his nose, waving his hands beside his ears to get my attention. I thought of the performances he and Nick put on for Del and me, dancing, singing, acting out comedies they created on their own, sometimes slap-stick, always fantastic and so well orchestrated.

I stared at Micah's empty bed, waiting.

The confusion and frustration of the last two weeks were a blur, filtering in and out as I searched my mind for answers to unanswerable questions. Del paced the floor, barely saying a word, only stopping now and again to look out the window. My mother made an attempt at small talk, biding her time, sweating it out until we heard a thump against the door, the thump of a wheel as it maneuvered to gain access. Tom slipped out as Micah was chauffeured back into the room, promising to return as soon as he heard anything in the way of test results. Still groggy, Micah accepted the surgical aide's help into bed and slept while five weary faces watched his every breath.

The steady beep, beep of the pump delivering Micah's IV saline solution became the focus of my attention. Methodical, rhythmic, and from rhythmic to primal. From somewhere deep inside came the sound of a drum, a hollow, earthy beat that thrummed in my brain. I saw myself seated around a campfire pit far away from the hospital on a plateau in the Grand Canyon (a place I loved). People were dancing; everyone was praying. Micah's room transformed, linoleum to rich dark earth, drywall became Redwall, tall, unencumbered limestone, extending upward as far as I could see. The only light was that of the stars and then the moon -- pulsating, reeling, responding to the beat -- to the ceremony -- to the call for healing, the healing of my son. There was nothing else. I felt my body react to the call of the drum -- swaying to the rhythm, moving with the beat.

Someone touched my shoulder. Within an instant, I was back -- no earth beneath my feet, no canyon walls, secure and protective -- only linoleum in a white sterile box of a room. It took a minute to refocus, to let the hospital settle in. Del's hand was on my back. Dr. Feusner was knocking on the door. "May I see you both?" Tom was with him.

"We'll wait with Micah, won't we, Grandma Nellie, Auntie Carol, Katy?" Tom's face wore a strained smile as he sat beside Grandma Nellie on the window seat. "He'll probably be sleeping for quite a while yet," he said.

My legs would not move. I knew, for better or worse, this was it. Del took my hand and led me down the hall to the now familiar conference room.

The same long table was strewn with the same bunch of papers. "Please, sit." Dr. Feusner motioned. His brow was furrowed, the lines around his eyes darker, more pronounced. It was the first sign of anything tangible I had seen on his face since we'd arrived. "Mrs. Chase. Mr. Chase," he said carefully, "Micah's bone marrow showed something we call Auer rods."

Slow motion. The words seemed to be rolling out of Dr. Feusner's mouth in slow motion.

"What that means, I'm afraid, is that he has leukemia."

"No...no!" I felt detached. Was my head missing? Were my feet? My heart left my body the moment Dr. Feusner

23

opened his mouth to speak, I was sure. I glanced at Del, who looked as pale as I felt, and then back at Dr. Feusner. "It can't be! There must be a mistake!" I said, breathlessly.

"Micah has none of the classic symptoms. Acute lymphocytic leukemia is what we most often see in children. What Micah has is acute myelocytic leukemia. AML is more commonly seen in adults. Micah's leukemia is associated with a condition known as Myelodysplastic Syndrome. Only approximately five percent of children diagnosed with acute myelocytic leukemia present initially as Micah has, with myelodysplastic syndrome."

This is bad." I pushed myself hard in order to concentrate. "This is really bad, isn't it? What do we do?"

"We feel it is vitally important to be aggressive with Micah's treatment. We would like to start chemotherapy immediately. Tomorrow, if possible." He reached for a stack of consent forms and handed them to me. "This protocol, called DCTER, is considered a study. That means we're still learning about this particular regimen of drugs and the effect they have as far as accomplishing remission."

Images on the consent forms flashed through my mind. I glanced at Del, hoping he would catch the important bits of information that were shooting past me at the speed of light.

"Take some time, read through the pages. I'll come back in a few minutes and explain anything you don't understand."

"Dr. Feusner, what are his chances with and without this treatment?" Del asked.

I shot Del a look. How dare he ask that question? Whatever the answer, I did not want to hear it.

24

There was another pause, this one feeling more torturous than the first: sweat beaded on my brow, I felt the blood drain from my face. "On the protocol," Dr. Feusner continued, "Micah has perhaps a sixty percent chance for survival. Without the chemotherapy, I'm afraid it would only be a matter of months. We could sustain him on transfusions for awhile, but it would only be a matter of time. I'm sorry."

Only a matter of months.

I stared at the stack of papers in my hands, oblivious to any remnants of conversation that took place. When Dr. Feusner left the room, I read each of them, one by one, and as I finished I passed them to Del. As the pages progressed, the content became more difficult to swallow. I felt myself slipping, sliding through the barrage of medical terminology. My ability to concentrate was coming and going, in and out, in and out, my brain taking in only as much information as I could handle at one time. When Micah's blood counts raised enough after the previous round, they would give him chemotherapy again. And again. And again. He would experience nausea, vomiting, weight loss and hair loss, not to mention the possible toxic effects to his heart, liver, and kidneys.

Dr. Feusner came back into the room. "I wish I had better news," he said. "I know this is difficult. Do you have any more questions? Is there anything I can do for you right now?"

"Micah, I've got to see Micah," I demanded, while signing the last of the forms. I'd had enough. This was someone else's world -- not Micah's, not mine, not Del's, or Nick's. It took everything I had to hold my tongue. What I wanted to do was scream, scream at all of them! The doctors. The nurses. All of them.

Chapter 4

Micah asked the same question I had asked earlier. "This is really bad, isn't it?"

Dr. Feusner didn't stumble over the word like I might have: *leukemia.*

"Your doctors have a plan, Micah. We're going to get this thing, we are." I was sitting next to him at the head of the bed. Del stood beside us and Dr. Feusner was to our left, holding Micah's hospital chart.

Micah scooted closer to me, and I wrapped my arms around him. "What did I do, Mom? Did I do something to cause this?" He was trembling, and his breathing was unsettled.

"No, baby. You didn't do anything. We don't know...it's just something..." I could feel his heart pounding as he leaned against my chest. He squeezed my hand.

"Okay, but I'm going to get well, right?" Micah's sweet voice cracked under the strain, but still there were no tears. His questions that followed were sharp and to the point. He asked for details, and Dr. Feusner gave them to him.

Micah went into surgery at 7:00 a.m. the following morning. The plan was to insert a catheter through which they would administer his chemotherapy, a tube running from the vein in his neck down into his chest and to his heart. One long hour later, we were still sitting in the waiting room -- Del with his head resting in his hands, his knees holding his elbows, his elbows keeping his exhausted upper body from collapsing into a muddled heap in the middle of the floor; me, rocking trancelike, unable to swallow past the jumble of nerves in my throat.

Debbie finally poked her head in the door, motioning for us to follow her. Del and I walked down the hallway and into a supply room where we were given sterile masks, gloves, gowns, and booties to put on. The surgery unit was to our right through a set of double doors. Several beds lined the walls of the recovery room. Tiny bodies slept in various stages of consciousness. No discrimination here: black, white, brown and yellow lay side-by-side in a world in which they had no control, no one child being treated any differently than the next. Anxious parents sat beside their children, some teary, some somber, some in that other place you go when you can no longer deal with reality. Nurses in masks and gloves moved quietly from bed to bed, checking vital signs, monitoring progress. My emotion-worn eyes searched the room. My feet made soft, swishing noises as I crossed the floor in the cloth booties I had placed over my shoes. The gown I'd been asked to put on was too big, kept falling off my shoulders, clinging to my jeans. As I walked, passing each bed, each child, I imagined my own germs, circling around my nose and mouth, kept there by the mask I wore to help ward off the spread of some unwanted organism within that sterile environment. I found it difficult to breathe with it on.

Micah's bed was on the far side of the room. His sheets

28

were stained with the yellow color of Betadine. So still; he was lying so still. Anxiety pushed the blood through my heart at a rate that made me woozy. I leaned over, took a deep breath, and stroked Micah's forehead.

He looked like an angel with his soft brown hair curling around his face. Needing to see, I gently pulled on the sheet covering his chest. My stomach cramped. I reeled, struggling to stay upright. "*Hold on, hold on*," I told myself. "*He needs you to be strong.*"

Micah's perfect little chest was now patched with gauze and tape. Two thin white tubes with caps on each end protruded out about eight inches past where they exited his body. I knew, yet there was no way I could have been prepared. Intrusive. This whole thing was intrusive. I closed my eyes and shook my head, hoping to clear things up, to find myself at home, out by the garden, watching Micah play basketball by the garage. No luck. I was still there, and so was Micah, hooked up to a heart monitor with a catheter inserted into his chest.

Over the days that followed, I rarely left Micah's hospital room, other than to use the restroom or grab something to eat on the run. I sat beside his bed watching for any sign of discomfort, for any need left unmet. Day turned to night; night was the same as day. More tests. People coming and going. Lights. No sleep. The smells. The air or lack of it. It was all the same.

Without realizing it, I took on an alternate role, that of a full-time nurse and advocate. I learned to monitor his IV pump, check his bag of fluids, and keep track of the medications he received. I started a journal, noting dates, times, drug schedules, and drug reactions. Sleep became Micah's main source of relief from the side effects of the chemotherapy. He was given anti-nausea drugs, but they were minimally effective. When he was awake, he tried to eat, but couldn't. Nothing tasted good; the smells of certain foods caused him to gag. It was hard to watch his refusal of grilled cheese, baked chicken, blueberry muffins, and tapioca pudding, things he usually loved.

Micah had always been a good eater. He liked most everything -- fruits, vegetables, meat and dairy. When we went out for dinner, he perused the salad bars, eagerly choosing his favorites from among the selections. While pacing the halls at the hospital, learning the routine, Del discovered that we could buy meals from the cafeteria downstairs, choices that were different from the usual hospital faire. There was even a salad bar with a wide variety of toppings: various veggies, cheeses, raisins, nuts, and shredded beef. Encouraged by Micah's enthusiasm, we foraged the buffet, loading a Styrofoam tray with items he would have chosen.

When Micah looked at the food, he grimaced. He could not eat more than a bite or two of the salad we so carefully put together. "I can't," he said. "Take it away, please." He held up his hand, gazing at the salad through the corner of his eye. He gagged and coughed. It hit me with the force of a plunging ocean wave: there was nothing I could do, no treat I could offer that would make any difference -- it was no longer up to me what meals were cooked, how food was served, if Micah ate or not. For twelve years it had been my responsibility to care for, nurture, and love my son. It was my job to make sure he ate nutritious meals each day, to

30

reassure him if he was feeling blue, to comfort him if he was ill. This was the first time in my experience as a mother that I felt helpless and at odds with my instincts.

Nurse Debbie affirmed my sense of loss. "Shelley, you're starting the grieving process," she told me that day. "You're grieving the loss of your healthy child."

I couldn't comprehend the rationale behind her words. *Starting the grieving process* meant something entirely different in my emotionally drained brain. I argued with her. "Don't tell me that," I said. "Micah's going to be fine! I'm not *grieving* my child."

Micah was scheduled to stay in the hospital for another two weeks. The hospital staff had been more than accommodating by allowing both Del and me to stay, but it had been two weeks since he was admitted. With our family and friends visiting often, the room had been a busy place. Space was at a premium. Between the window seat and a chair beside Micah's bed, naps had been taken, meals were shared, tears had flowed, but the inevitable could be put off no longer. Del needed to get back to work. Nick had been staying at his Auntie Jan's; that was good, but he needed to be at home, with one of his parents, at least.

On one of Del's trips around the hospital, he found an outside sitting area, a little oasis in the center of the hospital grounds. He told Micah about the huge oak tree that grew there, that there was a lawn and flowers, a fountain, blue sky. It gave Micah something to look forward to, a wheelchair ride maybe, when he was able. Del insisted I go there with him on the morning he was due to leave, reciting every reason he could think of: "We need to talk out of earshot from Micah. You need to get out of that room for

31

awhile. You'll know how to get to this place when Micah gets permission to go outside," he said, finally convincing me.

Even though I knew Del was right, walking away from Micah's room felt as if I was courting disaster. What if the next code blue was for him? I had heard the alarm, seen the blue light flashing, the horror on the faces of parents as they were shuffled out of their child's room by doctors and nurses rushing in from every direction; I'd seen a father huddled against a wall in the hallway, fearing the worst as a team of doctors performed extreme measures trying to keep his son alive; I'd heard a mother's anguished cry when the emergency resuscitation efforts on her daughter failed.

What if I wasn't there and something went wrong? What if Micah was alone and had an allergic reaction to his medication, if the stress of chemotherapy was too much for his heart, if he simply felt overwhelmed, and had no one to talk to? Del and I sat on a cement bench in the hospital gardens, looking up the side of the mountainous cement building, counting floors and windows, trying to locate Micah's room, to protect him from a distance. Our minds were on alert, but our thoughts were muddled. It took every ounce of self-control I had to keep from jumping up and running back inside. It was the first time I had been out of the building since we had arrived, the first time I had left Micah alone for more than a few minutes. We sat on the bench, discussing little things that needed to be done at the house, watering plants, caring for the animals, which bills needed to be paid. Neither of us could speak of anything more solid than that. I told Del that I would call every night, to keep him updated and to talk with Nick. I

32

asked him to hug Nick for me, to tell him how much I missed him, and that Micah and I would be home soon.

We walked back inside, past children hospitalized in the burn unit, rooms filled with kids suffering kidney problems, orthopedic maladies, heart and lung disease, cancer, sickle-cell anemia, HIV, and it struck me then that this hospital world was the real deal. For the families of chronically or terminally ill children, each day rested on decisions that were giving life and taking it away. The visiting hours for parents weren't such that they could go home to a routine of work and school and play and a good night sleep. Cancer therapy didn't stop for Cub Scouts or ballet lessons, soccer games, or pep rallies. We were now the parents of a very sick child. Our daily schedule would include blood draws and Broviac care, wearing surgical masks when Micah's counts were low. We would be in and out of the hospital, traveling to Oakland on a regular basis. Nick would miss out on so many things, and there would be little normalcy to Micah's life. I wondered if he would experience adolescence in any sense of the word?

This was no daydream. It wasn't a cruel joke. There was no misdiagnosis. It was real.

As we walked into Micah's room, a bell rang, and rang again, announcing an empty bag of antibiotics. Micah woke up, rubbing his eyes. "Hey," he said, his smile turning to a frown as his thoughts were interrupted, as nausea gained control.

Del gave Micah a goodbye hug. "Be good to these nurses, okay? Don't give them too much trouble."

"Who me?" Micah said, grinning sideways past the distress in his stomach.

33

After Del left, Micah and I got busy with a game of Yahtzee. We called my sister, Micah's Auntie Jan, to see if she could bring Nick to the hospital for a visit soon.

The following morning, Auntie Jan and Uncle John brought Nick, Grandma Nellie, cousins, Levi and Season, to see Micah. Apparently, as they entered the hospital lobby, they were questioned by security. "What floor?" the guard asked.

"Fifth, please," Jan told them.

"No young children are allowed on the fifth floor," the security guard said.

"But my nephew is a patient up there. This is his brother and these are his cousins."

"It's for the patient's protection, you understand. There are a lot of kids up on the fifth floor with compromised immune systems. It's hospital policy that young children wait here, in the lobby."

Jan phoned Micah's room. The news she gave was understandable but unexpected. It was another reality check for all of us. John stayed with Season and Levi. Nick was allowed to come up with Jan and Grandma Nellie, but he had been asked to put on a surgical mask. He walked over to Micah's bed and touched Micah's arm. Micah grinned at him. "Hey," he said to Nick. "Cool face-gear."

"Hey," Nick said. "Yeah, I know. They made me put it on." Nick backed away, came and sat on my lap.

Jan stood at a distance. None of us were sure now how close they should be, how easily Micah might contract some unbeknownst bug. Even Micah backed away slightly, leaning against his pillow, his arms wrapped protectively around his chest.

"What cha been doin'?" Micah asked Nick.

"Nothin'," Nick said.

"You feedin' Butchy for me?"

"Yeah."

"Oh, man, Nick, you should see the video game cart they have here! It's got everything! Mario Brothers, Zelda, Duck Tales, Contra, Double Dragon."

"Can we play?" Nick walked to Micah's bedside, rubbed the bedspread with his fingers.

"I don't know. Mom?"

"I'll see if I can find the cart."

Thank God, I thought. Some things never change. Tears filled my eyes as I watched my boys visit. Their bond as brothers quickly bypassed any barriers that had been placed between them by hospital regulations. They were happy just to be in the same room. Children have the magical ability to go on despite the odds, and it was no different for Micah and Nick. There was evidence of this everywhere around me. Down the hall, it was someone's birthday; a little girl with beautiful blonde curls sat with her family in the playroom, her smiling face covered in chocolate. Another little girl, around three, peddled her way up and down the hall on a pink and white Hot Wheels car, stopping to have a chat with a nurse now and again. Micah's bed was always littered with school books, pads of paper. At home, he had worked out on his weight bench every day and since he could not do that in the hospital, he had asked Del to bring his hand weights, at least, the next time he came to visit.

Auntie Jan moved closer to Micah's bed. Her feet moved like feathers as she crossed the floor. Her voice was no louder than her feet had been. "I love you," she said. Her words were as a breath of air exhaled during sleep -- that light, that quiet. "Last night on the Me-Wuk reservation, back home," she explained, "a Me-Wuk Grandfather sang and prayed for you. He made this medicine bag by hand. Inside it he put his tribe's special medicine, some sage and cedar, and the small heart-shaped stone you keep on your dresser." Micah looked at her, wide-eyed. "There's also a tiny quartz crystal in here and a sea shell you found in Monterey." Auntie Jan placed the medicine bag around Micah's neck.

Debbie came in carrying a bag of platelets for Micah. He clutched the leather pouch, explaining its importance with vivid animation while Grandma Nellie, Jan, and I sat on the window seat watching his hands, his eyes, keep the medicine bag alive through the telling of its tale.

Micah was a natural at storytelling. Every night, as he grew up, we told stories at bedtime. Once a week, we had 'our time', when the boys would snuggle with me in bed and ask for their favorites, some that I made up, others that were real, like about the day they each were born: "Nick, you were a contented little guy from the start," I would say. "You took your time, didn't want to be rushed. You were born with a smile on your face, never fussy, always happy. And Micah, "He's a keeper!" the doctor said, when he first saw you. It was in the middle of a blizzard, the worst snow storm in years. Your dad and I plowed our way down Big Hill Road in a 4-wheel-drive Jeep. You were determined even then to let the world know you were coming."

"All ready," Debbie said, interrupting my reflection. She checked Micah's blood pressure, took his temperature, and adjusted the plastic line delivering his platelets. By the time she left the room, the effects of the Benadryl she had administered seemed to be taking effect. Micah rubbed his eyes and yawned, waving goodbye to Nick, Grandma Nellie, and Auntie Jan as they stood in the doorway, ready to leave. Nick seemed hesitant; he turned back and stared at Micah as if waiting for him to say something, do something; he was accustomed to his brother having the last word, sending him off with a wish-you-well or a joke.

A bag of platelets the color of grapefruit juice hung from Micah's IV pole, dripping their way into his blood stream. He was groggy and trying hard to stay focused. "Why don't you ring the damn doorbell?" he said, momentarily confused.

"Micah!" I giggled.

Nick smiled and chuckled the same deep belly laugh he had laughed since he was a baby. From the time he was little, his favorite diversion had been his brother. It didn't matter if Nick was teething or had an earache, if dinner was late, or if the world seemed topsy-turvy, as long as Micah was in the room making faces or acting silly. In the hospital room that day, purposeful or not, Micah had given Nick what he needed to be able to say goodbye.

An attendant came through the door with Micah's dinner. Micah inched over a bit, making room for me on the bed. "A little confused, are we?" I teased, running my fingers through his hair. Soft brown strands hung loose in my hand, hair that should be attached, hair that had already lost its life, its shine, was cadaverous now in appearance and feel. The spot on Micah's scalp from which it came appeared naked and white. "Micah," I said, startled.

37

"Mom, it's okay," Micah said, shrugging his shoulders. My protector, always. He smiled. "Let's shave it," he said. "Shave it bald."

"You'd like that wouldn't you," I teased, "to have your head like L.L. Cool J's…oh, brother." I laughed, and phoned the nurses station. Debbie responded immediately with a pair of electric clippers. "You have one great kid here, Mrs. Chase," she said, as she handed me the clippers.

Micah and I spent the next day playing checkers, reading books, watching a little television. Around eight o'clock in the evening, a tall, thin woman with short, dark hair poked her head in the door of Micah's room. "I hope you don't mind, but I wanted to come by and introduce myself." Her smile was genuine, her eyes, warm bays of trust amidst the wide sea of hospital confusion. "I'm Barbara Beach," she said.

"Hello," I said. "Please, come on in."

Dr. Beach shook my hand, and sat down on the bed next to Micah. "So, you're Micah Chase," she said, extending her hand to him. "I've been looking forward to meeting you.

I've heard you keep the nurses on their toes around here."

Micah smiled. "I try my best," he said.

"Well, now I understand why the entire fifth floor nursing staff has been fighting over who gets you as a patient." She smiled. "I work in the Oncology Clinic, so once you're out of here, and when you come in for monthly check-ups, I get to be your Doc. Is that cool?"

"Yeah," Micah said, "that's cool." His grin lit the room, along with my face. I whispered her name, *Dr. Barbara*

Beach, mentally tucking it away, realizing that she was to become our lifeline between hospital and home. My eyes held her with a frayed and needy gaze, stinging slightly as they pooled with tears. I mentally dogged her steps as she walked out the door and down the hall. Finally, I thought. Someone we can talk to. Someone who might help me make sense of all this.

I had two Jan's in my life, one being my sister, the other a longtime friend named Jan Lekas. The second Jan and I met in a high school typing class, had experienced many 'firsts' together, like boyfriends, final exams, dragging McHenry Boulevard in the Zukalmobile (my parent's 1957 Chevy station wagon), drinking Bacardi Rum mixed with Coca Cola, proms, break-ups, graduation. We went to different colleges but stayed in touch, talking about the men in our lives, protest marches in the 1960's, world events, rock concerts we had attended. Our occasional get-togethers became adventures, backpacking trips in the Sierra Nevada Mountains with our dogs. Jan was the maid of honor at my wedding. She loved my children as if they were her own.

Jan lived in Alameda, not far from the hospital, and regularly surprised Micah with treats, something she thought might tempt him into eating, like pizza, ice cream, frozen yogurt. She brought books and magazines, games she bought at the Nature Store. On the 4th of July, she brought Micah a cupcake with a candle and a small flag, hoping to lift his spirits on a day she knew it would be hard for him to be indoors. After she left, Micah and I watched from the picture window as people in the streets waved sparklers, shot off fireworks, celebrated Independence Day. We told stories, remembering years past, good times at Uncle Dave's house with family and friends, swimming, barbequing, ooing and awing as fireworks filled the night sky. I heard him sigh and knew he was missing his brother and his cousins, wondering if they had Piccolo Pete's, Snakes, Spinners, the Smoking House, what the grand finale would be, and if they were thinking of him, so far away in his hospital room.

The following week, Micah was allowed to take a walk around the hall. Wearing his mask and pushing his I.V. pole, we visited a classroom set up for the kids on the 5th floor. The room had computers and desks and was staffed with a part-time teacher. She offered Micah a chair. "No thank you," he said. "I'm finished with the work my teacher sent but maybe another time." She smiled, and told him to let her know if he needed anything. "Paper, pencils, anything," she said. As we continued our lap around the hall, we found the Teen Lounge, a room where teens could gather, talk, and play games. Micah took it all in, but chose not to interact. He was not ready to acknowledge that he would be involved with the hospital long enough to participate. It was easy to go along with and understand his denial as I was feeling the same way.

After four weeks of being in the hospital, it was time to go home. I had the paperwork, the latest lab results, had turned Micah's blue insurance card over to all the appropriate people to be swiped and documented for hospital billing. I had gone through and inventoried the two large boxes of catheter supplies we had been given by the hospital pharmacy. I'd had detailed training on how to

40

care for Micah's Broviac. Any germ that found its way into the catheter could cause serious problems, infections, or worse. Wearing sterile gloves, working off a sterile pad filled with gauze, tape, alcohol pads and Betadine swabs, antibiotic ointment, Heparin, and syringes, Debbie showed me how to clean and redress the insertion site, change caps and flush the catheter lines with Heparin. I practiced giving injections by shooting water into oranges. Micah thought it was hilarious, watching my hand shake as I plunged the syringe into the round fleshy fruit. He had made a friend, a boy named Maurice, who would tease and taunt me: "Come on Mama, jab that sucker! It won't bite ya. Stick it!" Maurice came all the way to Oakland from Nevada every couple of months for his cancer treatments. He walked with crutches and was not in isolation. On a trek down the hall one day, he noticed Micah sitting on the edge of the bed and came in the room to say hello. "I'm Maurice. I got bone cancer in my leg. What you got?" he asked.

"I've got leukemia," Micah told him, a bit apprehensively. It was the first time he had said it out loud. I saw him bite his lip and look away.

"Bummer," Maurice replied, shaking his head. "I know a kid just died from that." Micah and I reacted the same way, staring at each other in shock. "What's your name? Maurice asked.

"Micah."

"Well, Micah, we're gonna be good friends, that's for sure. I been here awhile, so I can give you the skinny on what's up and what's down, you know?"

Maurice visited Micah every day. They played cards,

41

Micah's Game Boy, the video games on the game cart, and they made up the Imagine Game: *"Imagine we're at a Giants game. Imagine we've been given tickets to a Bon Jovi concert! Imagine a Big Mac with cheese!"* He and Micah compared stories, discussing which nurses were best and complaining about one particular doctor who had a discouraging bedside manner and whom they had nicknamed *Dr. Doom and Gloom.* They quipped about being poked, the chemotherapy, and how it made them feel. "Like crap," Maurice said.

"Yeah," Micah agreed. "I sure don't feel like eating a burger and fries anymore."

After watching me attempt to poke Micah instead of my orange, watching me grimace and flinch, Maurice told Micah: "You're mom's cool. I wish I had her lookin' out for my bacon around here. She sees everything. You're lucky, man."

"Just do it, Mom! Jeez!" Micah said, holding his thigh just above my proposed injection site. I closed my eyes and let the needle find a home in the soft flesh of Micah's thigh, injecting the medicine I would have to give him twice a day once we got home.

Chapter 5

A thin, pale child with large dark circles under lashless eyes greeted Del as he came to pick us up. A blue mask covered Micah's nose and mouth. I could almost see the smile beneath it when he walked out the door and into the corridor. "Hey big guy, how's the pitchin' arm?" Del asked.

"Probably pretty rusty, Dad." Micah looked up and into Del's face as pools of liquid threatened to spill from his exhausted eyes.

"Why the mask?" Del asked.

"He's neutropenic," I said, smiling at Micah. "The chemo did its job. His blood counts have bottomed out.

"I've got no white blood cells," Micah added. "So no kissin' the girls for awhile, I guess."

Micah would have nothing to do with waiting in his room while Del loaded the suitcases and his Broviac supplies in the elevator. "I'm out-a-here," he said. "I wanna go home." At Debbie's insistence, he rode in a wheelchair to the hospital lobby, where we waited until Del brought the car around. The air outside seemed so fresh. Even in the heart of the inner city with the thick smell of exhaust, it was easier to feel alive and whole again. It was hot, August hot, but the heat was intoxicating after weeks in a sterile environment with only a degree or so of change to give a hint as to the shifting of seasons. Micah sounded short of breath as his lungs struggled to adjust. I was on high alert, aware of every sound, each involuntary crease of his brow that might suggest any discomfort.

The ride home was surreal. In Sonora, cars filled both lanes on South Washington Street. People were walking through town, going about their daily lives as if nothing had happened, as if nothing had changed. But everything had changed; we were living on some other level of consciousness, aware of bugs and germs and the slightest rise in Micah's body temperature. We stopped at the gas station to fill up. Micah got out of the car, still wearing his mask. A woman with a small child saw him and pulled her child away to another aisle of gas pumps. A man walking by took a wide birth, swinging far out of his way to avoid close contact. I could not believe what I was seeing but tried to ignore it, not wanting to call Micah's attention to their behavior.

Out of Columbia, Del turned onto Big Hill Road, and the smell of buck brush made Micah sneeze. A rooster crowed from somewhere nearby. I became hypnotized by the scenery until movement in the back seat caught my attention. Micah was fidgeting, maneuvering his seat belt over the catheter under his shirt. I bit my lip and clenched my jaw, forcing away any thoughts of the illness that was eating away at him. He could be tough. He had shown tremendous strength thus far and would continue to do so. I knew that about him. He was headstrong and confident. In our past life, I had joked about his stubborn streak, the way he worked on a project until it was done to *his* satisfaction. What a blessing, I thought to myself; being

44

stubborn and sturdy and strong, those where characteristics Micah would need in the coming months.

Dr. Feusner had explained that a side effect of the chemotherapy would be a 'fuzzy feeling', and I wondered if Micah was feeling that now. The air around me shifted, became stifling. My skin temperature rose from cool to warm, and I felt clammy in less than a second. My face beaded with moisture, my body prickled from head to toe. *Hate* is an emotion my sisters and I were taught as children to avoid. We could dislike something, we could disagree with someone, but *hate* was not a word that was used in our family, nor was it an emotion that was encouraged. Yet I *hated* a disease that until six weeks ago, I had never considered as an immediate threat, a disease with symptoms far removed from my safety zone. I *hated* the medicine that caused Micah's mental confusion, the orange bag of poison meant to cure his leukemia, and the lying still in a hospital bed and being awakened all hours of the night, and the noises, and the smells, and the constant infusion of new terminology, treatment plans with numbers instead of names. Micah's study was called CCG 2891 and was the treatment plan for children less than twenty-one years of age with newly diagnosed acute nonlymphoblastic leukemia. It required the administration of five drugs: Daunomcin, VP-16, Ara-C, 6-Thioguanine, and Decadron over four days. The timing of the second course would be determined by 'randomization' -- like flipping a coin -- the study read. *"If your child shows a response to the first cycle of treatment, a second identical cycle of treatment will be given two-three weeks later."*

No one would ever know how much I had wanted to

45

grab Micah and run away from the Children's Hospital, to take him home so he could be with his friends and his brother and his dog -- to be a normal kid again. Normal kid. The words bit at my ears. My entire life, I had been told that I was easy going, that I was calm in the face of a crisis, displaying composure and sensibility when drawn upon to provide care on any level. As we pulled into our driveway, as the goats bleated and the donkey brayed, as our home came into view and Nick bounded out the front door, I doubted those abilities more than I ever had before.

The car door was barely open before Butchy jumped in and was on Micah's lap, yipping and licking, turning back and forth between the front seat and the back as if he could not make up his mind which person he needed to greet first. "Did you miss me, boy? Did you miss me?" Micah asked. He made a pouch in his t-shirt and placed Butchy inside, cradling him the way he had done since Butch was a small puppy.

Nick, along with Del's parents, Dolores and Henry, waved from the porch. I had phoned from the hospital and told them what the doctors recommended regarding minimal contact. Micah would have to forego hugs until his white blood cells numbered high enough to provide him some immunity. Inside the house, welcome banners and balloons decorated the living room. Beautifully wrapped packages covered the hearth. "Is it somebody's birthday?" Micah asked as we walked through the door.

"It's your unbirthday," Grandma Dolores said, blowing him a kiss. "Welcome home."

Nick came over and touched Micah's shoulder, tentative, afraid it might hurt. Micah turned and smiled, punching Nick playfully in the arm. "Hey," he said. "Did you miss me?"

"Ya," Nick said. "I did."

The boys spent a moment looking at each other, taking stock of the changes they both had gone through. It was as if Nick needed to make sure Micah was still Micah, and Micah needed to make sure Nick thought of him that way.

Their relationship as brothers was unique to kids who are raised out of the mainstream. They had Chris and Caitie Deatsch, who lived down the street as playmates. The rest however, came to the house on weekends mostly, after initiating conversations and transportation with their parents. We lived five miles from the elementary school, ten miles from town. Families living on Big Hill were scattered, enjoying the space and security of mountain living. I did childcare after school most days for Chris and Caitie, friends Erik, Jessica, and Eli, but mostly, Micah and Nick relied on each other as companions. Though they occasionally fought like brothers do, they were very close. When they were small, Micah desperately wanted a room of his own. When he was five and Nick was three, we remodeled the house and built their two bedrooms side-by-side. We took their bunk beds apart and put one bed in each room. Micah was into Transformers and Ninja Turtles, and his room reflected that. Nick loved Ninja Turtles too, but he also loved Legos, Dinobots, and most things Disney. Micah collected geodes and baseball cards; Nick collected fossils, baseball cards, and bugs. They both loved seashells and had shelves filled with books. For at least a year after their move to separate bedrooms, I would go into Micah's room in the morning and find Nick on the floor beside him with his blanket and pillow and a stuffed animal or two. At first I thought Nick was initiating the switch, but later discovered it was Micah who would jiggle Nick on the shoulder in the middle of the night, help him carry his bedding, Care Bear, and bunny blanket to the floor beside Micah's bed.

One winter, after a heavy snow, Micah and Nick built an 'igloo' in our yard. They worked side-by-side, digging and stacking, convinced they could get the igloo done before it got dark, and if they did, that Del and I might let them spend the night in it. "We'll wear warm coats," Micah told me. "We'll have a flashlight," Nick added, hopefully. I smiled, letting the boys have their fantasy and continue their play. They worked all morning and into the afternoon until the mound of snow actually resembled an igloo. I checked on them occasionally, amazed by their perseverance. Micah sent Nick to the house to get me at one point, wanting to know how to 'build' a door. I put on my coat, gloves, and boots and helped them scoop snow until we had a good sized hole dug into their mound. We put boards on both sides of the hole to act as braces, and when Del got home from work, he used our snowplow to push a huge pile of snow up to the igloo and helped us complete the entrance into the snow cave. By four in the afternoon, the kids had had enough. They were content with the finished product, deciding that if they ever moved to Alaska they could now build their own house. Sleeping in the igloo never came up again. Both of them were happy with the hot lasagna I had made for dinner and snuggling beside me afterward, watching the fire pop in the fireplace while I read aloud a chapter from the *Hobbit*.

I emptied a large cabinet in the kitchen and filled it with Micah's Broviac supplies, bought a legal notepad to inventory and keep track of what we used and what we needed to order from the pharmacy. I also bought a new calendar, one with space enough to write notes each day to keep track of when we had done blood draws, what days we went to see Micah's local doctor, scheduled clinic visits to Oakland, and anything I saw as far as changes in Micah's condition.

For the first couple of days after we got home, Micah's dreams were haunted by the weeks he had spent at the hospital. His bed sheet became a tourniquet, binding his arms and legs as he thrashed about. He woke out of breath, unsure of where he was, frightened of the dark, crying out. As I rushed into the room, his hands groped for something familiar, searching for his nightstand, his bed lamp, making sure he was home -- *home* -- and not in the hospital. I could see him relax as I straightened his bedding, rubbed his back, lay beside him until he was sleeping soundly again. Lying there, I could feel his heart keeping time, beat for beat, with my own. Using the technique I had been taught during childbirth classes in the weeks before Micah was born, I slowed my breathing, relaxed my muscles, trying to reach him on a primal level, soothing his mind and his body by reestablishing that early connection. The sensation I felt was one of utter completeness on a level I had never experienced. If ever I could have passed healing energy from my body into Micah's it was then, at that moment of closeness in the deepest dark of night.

Micah seemed to thrive on my home cooking. The

49

color returned to his cheeks. As he began to feel better, he ate more, became more active. When his white blood cell count reached five hundred, the magic number that indicated his immune system was at a functioning level, that he was no longer neutropenic, his best friend, Jason, was allowed to come over for short visits. He brought Micah's homework, explaining the lessons he had missed at school, talking about who was going out with who, what their friends had done over the summer, and what was happening now in seventh grade. Jason's mother, Diane, would often come with him. Not only was she my friend, she was a licensed nurse, and while the boys visited, we would go over Micah's lab results and talk about the after-effects of the chemotherapy he was experiencing. During the day, while Nick and Jason were in school, Micah and I kept busy with his schoolwork, playing games, and taking short walks. It was time to think about my returning to work, so Micah and I brainstormed ideas about how he might manage if he needed to be home alone on some days. I talked with him about possibilities that might come up as far as fever and injury. We made a list of emergency phone numbers. Both of his grandmothers agreed to come as often as they could to keep him company and help with his care. My time away would not be easy, but it was necessary. We wanted to keep some semblance of normalcy in our lives, not only for Micah and Nick, but for Del and me as well, and since we lived paycheck to paycheck, both our salaries were necessary in order to cover our monthly expenses. In addition, a year earlier we had opted to drop the boys and I from the insurance policy Del carried through his work. My employee insurance package offered better coverage and paying monthly premiums on two policies amounted to salary deductions we couldn't afford. Since my policy was now our only source of insurance coverage for Micah, taking an unpaid leave of absence without benefits was not an option for us. The reality of our growing financial responsibilities, the importance of providing the kids with a healthy, balanced environment circled my brain constantly, but the thought of leaving Micah alone, shook the foundation of everything I believed in as a mother.

As parents, we take for granted the cycles of our children's lives: we watch them grow from babies to toddlers; we see them start school, move into adolescence, and then on to adulthood. There are established guidelines but no finite rules. We read books, listen to the advice of experts in the field. Mostly though, we proceed by gut instinct, encouraging, pulling back, holding on, letting go. This unexpected roadblock in Micah's life experience was a blind passage into a big black hole. The only rules we had were the ones in our gut, the only guidelines, those we made together as a family.

One morning, I woke up early, bundled up in my robe and slippers, and walked outside onto the deck. The sun was rising over the top of the Dardanelle Cones in the distance, trailing pink and orange fingers of light across the gray pre-dawn sky. Our view from the mountaintop stretched over a vast canyon, looking out on the rugged backcountry between Columbia and Twain Harte. The Dardanelle Cones stood like proud sentinels to the East, marking the top of Sonora Pass, an area we frequented when camping or picnicking. The Cones were like old friends as I had grown up in their shadows, attending

YMCA camp nearby, fishing at Clark's Fork with my parents and sisters, and playing alongside the river at Frasier Flat and Kennedy Meadows. I had taken Micah and Nick to those same places along with others we discovered over the years. On one particular trip, the three of us drove along Crabtree Road out of Long Barn, heading down to the Clavey River. Somehow, I got a little bit lost, turning on a forest service access road rather than staying on the main road down to the river. While I concentrated on my driving, the boys sang songs: "Wheels on the Bus," "Down by the Bay," the "Cannibal King." When Nick grew concerned, Micah calmed him, saying, "Don't worry, Nicky, we're not lost. We're just having an adventure." Since Nick was a baby, he had trusted his brother above anyone else. He and Micah had faith in each other, and both of them had faith in me. Even on an unpaved river road, through territory that was rough and unfamiliar, they knew I would take care of them and keep them safe.

Did that same truth hold now, I wondered sadly, staring at the familiar faces of the Dardanelle Cones? Could I guide my boys through the rough uncharted waters ahead, take care of them and keep them safe? A breeze blew through the pines, sending loose needles tumbling onto the deck. The perfume of cedar, an essence of sage, greeted me as I stepped onto the front lawn and walked toward my garden. I strolled down a neglected row of pole beans, left over from spring, hanging wilted and brown from their tee-pee like supports. The garden chairs were covered with debris, so I swept them off with my hand before sitting down to enjoy the morning, the peaceful trill of a morning dove, the love songs of the orioles. Micah came outside,

52

still in his pajamas, walked over and sat in my lap. He let me kiss the special place on his neck I called "my spot". At twelve years old, he was not supposed to like snuggling with his mom so much; sometimes in front of his friends, he pretended like he didn't, but the truth was he still did. I held him tight, both of us absorbing the tenderness of the moment for as long as it would last.

"Mom, I love you."

"I love you too, baby."

"Mom?"

"Yes?"

"I think I know what it feels like to die."

Was that a rip in my gut? "What do you mean?" I asked, fearfully.

"I think it feels soft, like angel wings." Micah looked into my eyes. "Do you think it hurts to die?"

My fragile existence cracked a little more. I had never given him reason not to hope. "Micah, we don't know..."

"I've been having dreams, Mom, about what it would be like, what it would feel like to die."

My rocking gained momentum. My grip on Micah grew tighter.

Three weeks after Micah's homecoming, he was readmitted into the hospital to begin his second round of chemotherapy. This second stay lasted another full month. Del and I rotated shifts -- I stayed three weeks with Micah, and then he stayed the last week. This rotation worked but was difficult to maintain. When at the hospital, I worried about Micah, but I also worried about Nick -- whether he was eating properly, getting his schoolwork done, if he was lonely or feeling sad. While at home, I stressed over what was happening with Micah at the hospital -- was he being cared for properly, was he hurting, was he scared. Del and I began communicating on a different level -- talking in circles, discussing issues but avoiding emotional pitfalls. We spoke by telephone several times each day, but it was impossible to relate the true state of our circumstances. At times, I felt as if I was talking to a stranger, someone technically vague and emotionally distant. Internalizing, as well as prioritizing, became a regular part of our routine. With Micah and Nick, our words were soft and real, but as a couple, we began floundering for moments of depth and understanding. Though we could probe the doctors for more information, listen intently to their every word, it seemed impossible to do that same thing with each other -- saying it out loud, as parents, made things too real, too immediate for us to handle.

At the end of November, immediately following Micah's third round of chemotherapy, an appointment was set to discuss the possibility of bone marrow transplantation. Del and I read the literature sent to us by the transplant center, staring at each other through hazy eyes, trying to grasp what this new step in Micah's treatment might mean for him, for us, as a family. When the day finally came, however, we were prepared to discuss Micah's options. The transplant team, consisting of two doctors and a nurse, met with us in a treatment room inside the transplant facility at the University of California Hospital at San Francisco. Dr. Calloway introduced himself and the others. "In Micah's case we are very limited, Mrs. Chase, Mr. Chase," Dr. Calloway told us. "I'm sure you know that

Micah has a very rare form of leukemia. It's quite possible he may not go into a remission."

Though I had resolved to be strong, my heart betrayed me. My chest heaved, seemed to have a mind of its own. Pools of tears that should have dried up long ago overflowed unchecked.

Dr. Calloway's nurse responded with a box of Kleenex. "But it's possible, isn't it? Are you telling us it's not possible?"

"No, not at all. But we need to go over Micah's options should remission not occur."

"A bone marrow transplant?" I asked.

"Yes. Micah has a brother, is that right?"

"Yes, Nick," I said.

"Good. Yes. Nick." Dr. Calloway made a note on Micah's chart. "Nick should be tested as soon as possible. You must know, however, there's only a one-in-four chance he inherited the same HLA molecules as Micah. If there were more siblings, the chances for a match would be greater. Unfortunately, that's just the way it works."

"What about Del and me?"

"Each of you, as Micah's parents, can only be a half-match. You'll still need to be tested to see which of you is a better candidate should the need arise. That scenario involves a different type of transplant, one we'll discuss later if necessary.

"For now, let's step back a bit. Let's say Nick isn't a match," Dr. Calloway continued. "Then using marrow from an unrelated donor would be the most likely scenario. Unfortunately, the chances of finding any two unrelated individuals with the same HLA markers vary widely. I understand you have some Native American ancestry?"

"Yes."

"That could make things more difficult. The pool of Native American donors is small."

"We have mixed ancestry. Del is part Irish, part English. I'm half Austrian, some English, French, and Choctaw Indian. Does that make a difference?" Beads of sweat formed on my brow, the blood drained from my face.

Dr. Calloway's nurse stood up, cleared her throat, and motioned to Dr. Calloway.

"Perhaps a glass of water, Mrs. Chase?" she said.

My head began to spin. Everything in the room looked a dingy brown color. Memories tumbled through my mind like shifting sand. I remembered Dr. Feusner talking about finding a perfect match, about blood types, a willing donor. I remembered that a neighbor's cat had contracted leukemia, was treated by the family veterinarian, and survived. I thought of a friend of Nick's whose sister committed suicide, how angry Micah got when he found out: "How could someone do that?" he shouted. "How could she give up her life like that when I'm struggling so hard just to survive?" I felt like a mad woman trapped in a world I did not want to be in.

"After receiving chemotherapy," Dr. Calloway was saying, "Micah will begin radiation treatments. He will have to be in isolation at this time for his own protection.

I pictured the Mother's Day card Micah wrote when he was nine years old: *"Mom,"* it read. *"I love u, I love u, I love u: you are a sweet, kind woman who swims, loves everybody, helps animals and kids, gives me first aid, drives my friends everywhere, hugs me a lot, kisses me a lot, is always cheerful and happy."* I sat tall

56

and took a deep breath, trying to live up to Micah's praise. Dr. Calloway was still talking.

"The actual transplantation of marrow is very simple, done in the manner of a normal blood transfusion. Healthy marrow cells travel through the circulatory system and somehow, miraculously, find their way to the bone cavities where they began to grow and reproduce on their own. Barring complications, Micah could be out of isolation in three to six weeks. Are you okay? Any questions?"

"Go ahead, please," I said, wearily.

"These protocols are all very new -- all are experimental. You'll need to be cleared by your insurance in advance to make sure a bed space can be held for Micah. When we're finished here, we'll send you to Greta in Admissions to get that process started."

"It sounds like you're telling us, any way things go, you're recommending a transplant."

"Yes, we are. In Micah's case, we are."

"So," Del interjected, "what do we do now?"

"You find as many people as you can to be tested for a possible match. You have donor drives. You spread the word."

"Okay," I said, stiffly. "Now give us the rest. If this possibility exists for Micah, I want to hear it all -- side effects, everything."

Dr. Calloway continued, describing isolation, transfusions, nutrition, mouth care, everything. Nasty bit by nasty bit, we heard it all -- infections, bleeding, liver disease. Rejection and relapse. There was Graft Versus Host Disease, a complication where the body's newly transplanted white blood cells attack the host cells -- the

57

patient -- causing symptoms that range from mild to severe rashes, jaundice, and diarrhea. Bacterial infections. Weight loss. Early and prolonged treatment with steroids -- Methotrexate, Prednisone, Cyclosporine.

Dr. Calloway stopped his description abruptly. Enough was enough. "I want you to spend some time talking with my nurse now about fund-raising, and recruiting. Testing donors can be expensive. You'll need some support." He offered his hand as did his silent partner.

Both men swished out of the room in their long white coats -- white coats -- for better or for worse, my family's world now consisted of a myriad of long white coats.

Dr. Calloway's nurse was a treasure trove of information and plans. Her ideas gave us a place to put our energy and a glimmer of hope on which to focus. She arranged for Del, Nick and me to be HLA tested at Oakland Children's Hospital. "What about my sisters and Del's siblings?" I asked. "Should they be tested?"

"Everyone can get tested," the nurse told us. "Aunts and uncles. Cousins. Let us know who's interested, and we'll make the arrangements. It's a good place to start."

Before we left we went to Admissions to turn in the insurance information. So far, everything had been covered by our healthcare plan. I anticipated no problems. Neither did Greta in Admissions.

From Micah's diary:

Sept. 12, 1991

"I want to go to school. My grandma's here, and I love her, but it's hard being home. Hopefully, pretty soon, I'll get to see my friends. I really miss them. Today my mom did a blood draw. She went to the hospital to drop it off before work. I hope the results are good. I really need them to be good."

Sept. 13, 1991

"My counts are better, but my skin around my Broviac got hurt somehow. It might be an irritation from the tape we use. Mom stayed home from work to fix it. I love my mom. My brother is going to bring my work home from school today. Mr. Larkin called to see if I needed any help with my algebra. He's a good teacher."

Sept. 16, 1991

"Today we did another blood draw. My grandma is here for the whole week. That really makes me happy. We had a great weekend. On Sunday we played golf. There was hardly anybody on the course, which was good for me, with my counts being low and all. We had so much fun! Afterward Dad took me for a ride on his motorcycle. Nice!"

Sept. 17, 1991

"Me and my brother had a water fight today. It was cool! I had to duck and cover because of my Broviac, but Nick was careful and aimed low (for once!)."

Sept. 23, 1991

"I finished my chemo last night. This morning I woke up with a

59

terrible headache. They gave me morphine to get rid of the pain. It wasn't just a headache; it was a reaction to the blood transfusion I had received. It hurt worse than anything yet. It scared me. I thought I was having an attack of some kind. I don't know why, but it hurt that bad.

"I feel like I'm on a rollercoaster, but not like the one at Santa Cruz where you want the ride to go on forever. On this rollercoaster, I want to get off. I want to hang out with Kip and I want to dream big: I want to get my driver's license and take Nick for rides in my Lamborghini. I want to build my mom a house on the beach and become a doctor and discover a cure for leukemia."

Sept. 24, 1991

"Today I woke up in my own bed, in my own house, and it felt great. Dr. Beach told me no more weekly bone marrow aspirates. Thank gosh! I'm feeling good. No hair, but that's okay. Dr. Beach says I look good even without hair. She's awesome. I'm really glad she's my doctor. She knows what I'm feeling and thinking. I can talk to her and I know she'll tell me the truth.

"My mom and I played the Imagine Game. I imagined I was flying. I imagined I was free. I imagined I was in remission."

Sept. 24, 1991

"This is my second day at home. I still can't go to school. Me and my grandma went golfing today. We had a good time. We took in a blood draw but my counts haven't come back yet. Hope they're good! Like my mom says, I'm trying to make lemonade out of lemons."

Sept. 25, 1991

"Today we played golf again. I didn't do very well. Something's

60

wrong with my leg. It scared me a little. It kind gave out from underneath me and I stumbled. It really hurt. We went to Taco Bell for lunch but I couldn't go in because I'm neutropenic. When we got home, my new teacher was there. She's a home school teacher and her name is Suzanne DeLacy. I'm really trying to keep up with my schoolwork and this will help a lot."

October 1, 1991

"I'm reading Behind the Cracked Mirror. *It's really good. It makes me want to write a book of my own. I love to read and I already write stories. I've been doing that since I was a little kid. My mom says I'm really good at it and my teachers have told me that too. I think I will do it. I will write a book someday.*

"Here's a story I wrote for Nick when I was 10 years old. I keep all the stories I write. This one makes me laugh. I was pretty young and some of the words are a little goofy, but I still like it. Suzanne wanted to read my old stories and she liked this one too, so I'm putting it here in my journal.

"Yesterday my brother and I discovered a cave. We decided we would come back later and explore it with the right clothes and with ropes. After we got home, I couldn't help myself. I got on my old pants and went back to the dark threatening cave. I turned my flashlight on. I stumbled in. I saw a turn ahead and walked slowly around the bendy passage. There in front of me was a beautiful lake! It was so beautiful it was almost imaginary! Little bugs glided along the surface. I could see them shimmering in the light. In my excitement, I forgot all about my parent's rule about safety first. I ran right into the water. It felt glorious. I dipped and bobbed, wishing my brother Nick was there.

All of a sudden, I saw the most hideous thing I've ever seen! It

61

was a bat! It had fangs and big yellow eyes! I swung my fist and whacked it away from me. I climbed out of the water, quivering with fear. I got out of the cave and headed straight for home. I went in the house and checked on Nick, making sure he was safe and asleep and that he hadn't followed me to the cave. He does that sometimes. When I finally lay down, I was so restless that I couldn't sleep. I decided that next time I'd bring Nick along, because he's my brother and together we can do anything."

"Bendy passage??? Ha!!! I think I'll rewrite this and maybe try to publish it.

"Mom took my blood work in and called me from school. I'm not neutropenic anymore. My ANC is 588!"

October 7, 1991

"Today we took in another blood draw. Last weekend I got to play with Jason both days. Mom took us to the 7-11 to play pinball and other games. It was great. I know how hard she tries to keep my life normal. And that's what I want. I appreciate it so much. I might get to go back to school in a week or two. Yeah!"

October 9, 1991

"I'm back in the hospital, for four days of chemo. I had a spinal tap. It didn't hurt very bad. Dr. Feusner's a pro. Home Monday? I hope."

Chapter 6

By the end of December, Micah had been in the hospital four times and finished four cycles of chemotherapy. Each stay lasted between three and four weeks, and he managed the majority of that time fairly well. The results of the bone marrow testing by family members had come up empty. No donor match. No donor. Del and I took in the information we were given regarding the individual test results, but only partly, as it was impossible to digest their full implication. Micah withheld his usual barrage of questions, choosing to side-step the issue of transplantation.

The doctors put Micah on a new medication for his nausea, and though his appetite was still poor, mealtime became more manageable. He could stomach chocolate ice cream and tapioca from the hospital cafeteria. He zestfully downed cartons of apple and cranberry juice and drank milk on occasion. He enjoyed eating bananas, peaches, and yogurt. He even managed chicken strips, corn, and a few bites of mashed potatoes. In the afternoons, if his counts were not too low, we would often cruise the hallway. Micah would push his portable IV pole, and I would struggle to keep up, futzing with the IV tubing when it got too close to the wheels. "Mom," he would say, jokingly. "This isn't rocket science. Just hold that tubing out of the way, and let's boogie."

Some days we would search out Maurice, if he hadn't yet swung into Micah's room on his crutches. The nurses would tie off their IV's and release them from the confines of their IV pole and pumps. We would find an extra wheelchair, and Maurice and Micah would have races down the hall, giggling, displaying the constitution of teenagers-to-be, despite their circumstances. The nurses spurred them on, encouraging the exercise. One lap, sometimes two and they were done, satisfied for the moment with the freedom they had been given.

A couple of times we were allowed a four-hour field trip to Jan Lekas's house, giving Micah a respite from the chemo routine and a little fresh air. Micah had to promise to keep his mask on, to stay away from people as much as possible. He was tired, but not too tired to tease Jan about her old Motorola television set and the fact that he had to turn the channels manually instead of using a remote control. Micah loved Jan Lekas. When he was two years old, she took him to the Oakland Zoo, where he rode on a giant tortoise, saw elephants, and alligators. Later that same day, Micah poked his head through the rod iron railing around Jan's stairs, and got stuck. He cried until we reminded him of the funny monkeys in the zoo, and then he laughed and made monkey noises, relaxing his muscles enough that we could pull him free.

Micah's 4th trip to the hospital was rougher than most. He'd had a bad reaction to a transfusion just before we were due to go home, got a fungal infection, and had to be put on Amphotericin, a medication known as 'Amphoterrible'

64

on the 5th floor at Oakland Children's. While on the medication, he shivered uncontrollably, his teeth chattered, his body ached. No amount of warm blankets or Benadryl seemed to help. I climbed up next to him on his bed, cuddling close, using my body heat to comfort him. Worried that we would not get to spend Christmas at home, the doctors and nurses worked doubly hard to make it happen, releasing Micah on December 21st.

Micah was weak and tired but anxious to set up the tree. The relief in Nick's eyes when I pulled out our box of decorations was telling; the thought of missing Christmas as a family had loomed heavily over all our heads until that moment when we strung the Christmas lights, hung our ornaments and placed the angel on top of the tree. The boys snuck around the house that night, conspiring to find their presents, looking in closets, cupboards, and under the beds. Every year they tried to outwit me and find their gifts. When they grew too close to my hiding place, I would shoo them away, and they would squeal and laugh, whispering to each other about some new scheme they had hatched.

The joy on their faces that Christmas morning was unsurpassed. Micah screamed and jumped up and down when he opened his vintage Willie Mays baseball card. Nick fired up his remote control car with equal enthusiasm. Both boys seemed as happy as ever.

Just after New Years, I got a call from Dr. Beach.

"Shelley, how's Micah feeling?" she asked.

"Great, I can't slow him down. He's eating like a horse. He looks great, a little pale, but great, why?"

"Shelley, Micah's blood-work showed a problem. We didn't get remission. I'm sorry."

I held tight to the receiver, feeling numb. Every waking hour, I had focused on convincing myself that the chemotherapy would work. Sitting in the dark, holding back a scream, I thought about how to tell Micah the news. As strong as he appeared, I knew he was scared. Sometimes I heard him pray late at night, asking God to take the leukemia away, to make him healthy and whole again, to let him live. In the car, on the way back home from the hospital, he would repeat a mantra: "I *will* get remission, I *will* get remission." He would always smile at me after with hope in his eyes. "Right, Mom?" he'd ask. "I *will* get remission."

"No doubt about it," I would tell him as hopeful as he.

I told Del, and we told Micah together.

In his room, on his bed, Micah shrugged his shoulders and called Butchy into his lap. He bit his lip to keep from crying. "That doesn't mean it isn't going to happen," he said, his voice cracking. Nick poked his head around the corner, and Micah motioned him to come in. "Don't worry," Micah told Del and me. "It will all be okay," he promised his brother.

Micah and Nick snuggled next to me in bed that night. We told stories in rounds. I started the story. Nick added to it and then Micah. By the time Micah took his last turn, Nick was asleep. Ending the story with, *"they lived happily ever after,"* Micah's voice sounded broken, raspy. I reached up and touched his cheek, moist with tears. I kissed him, held him tight. "Oh baby," I whispered, "let's try not to worry."

"I want to go to school," he whispered. "I want to see my friends."

Though Micah's attitude had remained positive throughout his time at the hospital, the isolation, the drugs, all of them together were beginning to consume his resolve. No matter which direction he turned, someone was checking his vital signs, testing his blood, counting his calorie intake, measuring his output. Even in his dreams, they did not let him rest, coming at him with needles the size of knives and putrefying medicines in little paper cups. It was humbling, humiliating, and he was getting tired of it.

If Micah was going to stay committed and strong, we had to loosen the strings. I talked with Dr. Beach, and the decision was made: as soon as his counts were up enough to feel safe after this last round of chemo, he could go back to school. His seventh grade teacher had arranged for a home tutor so he wouldn't fall behind, but that wasn't enough. Micah needed to be with his friends.

Every day, Nick brought Micah's homework home from school. Micah worked on his own in the evening and with his tutor in the afternoons. He talked with his friends on the phone and kept busy writing in his journal, taking short walks, playing Nintendo. His neutrophil count reached the magic number, 500, the following Friday. We celebrated by ordering pizza and renting a movie. By Sunday afternoon, he had his clothes laid out on his bed. Monday morning he was the first one up, showered and dressed, his backpack filled and waiting by the door.

Though the decision was the right one, it came with trepidation. I didn't know how the kids would react. Micah had no hair, no eyebrows, no eyelashes. It had been nearly five months since they had seen him. A lot had happened. When the day finally came, the problem took care of itself. Micah's teacher had prepared them ahead of time as to what they could expect, but it wouldn't have mattered if he hadn't -- they were all so happy to have him back, the issue of hair or no hair was no issue at all.

Micah's blood counts were frighteningly low a great majority of the time, so it was with a deep breath and a prayer that I sent him off to school each day wearing his baseball cap and a smile. He wouldn't accept anything other than to be treated normally. He wanted to be like any other kid, any one of his friends, to live a full and happy life. Basketball season presented a new challenge to everyone but him. Micah insisted on playing regardless of the myriad of protests he encountered. By this time, Dr. Beach knew better than to argue. He was the team's point guard, his position for the past three years. There was no way he was going to give it up. If it meant fighting for the position, he would do it.

Running the court, giving it everything he had, Micah played with unyielding determination. Not even his monthly visits to the Oncology clinic could stop him. The procedure he underwent was painful. Both a bone marrow aspirate and a biopsy were routine, but with the help of medication and his confidence in Dr. Beach, he never shed a tear. "Micah's the only kid I know," she would tease, "who can tell jokes while getting a three inch needle shoved into his backside." The nursing staff on those days bowed to his every whim. No messing around -- Micah had to be home by game time. I would watch him as he hobbled out to the car, another trip to the clinic over and done. Back at school, he would take a deep breath, and ready himself to walk into the gym, body stiffened, head held high, the posture itself an illusion he had created to cover up the intensity of the pain he felt. Was it his friends, I wondered, or himself, that needed convincing?

January 18th was Micah's birthday. He would be thirteen. His friends planned a surprise party. I oversaw the day's festivities with pain gnawing at my heart as I watched the other children, happy and healthy, the way Micah had been only a short time ago. While the kids danced and played video games, I sat on a stool at the kitchen counter, thinking, submitting for a moment to the rest my body so desperately needed. We were in a holding pattern as far as Micah's treatment. The pain of not knowing what would happen next was unbearable. The waiting was torture. It never went away, not even for a party. Dr. Beach was monitoring his counts and speaking weekly with the doctors at the transplant center in San Francisco. Since the best possibility of curing Micah's leukemia now meant a bone marrow transplant, the push to find him a donor had intensified. Micah's life now depended on the actions of a stranger, someone compassionate and mindful enough to walk through a clinic door somewhere and donate his or her bone marrow to save the life of a child they had never met. *All the peoples of this planet are members of the same human family,* my college anthropology instructor once told me. How could it be otherwise, when a total stranger could be a perfect bone marrow match for Micah, down to the finest detail of his genetic makeup? *"We found a match."* Oh, how I longed to hear those magic words.

Micah was on the recipient waiting list of the National Marrow Donor Program, a registry of donors worldwide. So far, there was no one on the list with genetic markers close enough to be his donor. The cost of testing potential donors was about $60.00 per person, and Heart of America, the California branch of the NMDR, generously offered to double any monies we could provide. Friends gathered together, making plans for a fundraiser and merchandise auction to help offset expenses.

The first obstacle to this impressive venture was pride. Financial obligations to the family, our children, was a parental responsibility Del and I would have to place in the hands of others if we were going to make this happen for Micah. It was difficult to admit that we needed help and to accept financial donations in lieu of managing by ourselves. More importantly, Micah did not want to go public with his disease, the painful struggle he had tried so hard to keep private. It took a lot of coaxing before he allowed a reporter to come to his basketball game, and then to our house for an interview.

The result of the newspaper article was an outpouring of support from the residents of Tuolumne County, California. Hundreds of people came to the fundraiser. Hundreds more came to the bone marrow drive to see if they were a match, giving their blood in hopes of saving Micah.

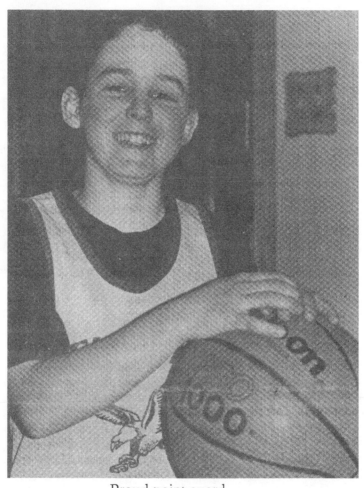

Proud point guard –
Micah Chase smiles after game

--used with permission of
The Union Democrat

The Union Democrat
Sonora, CA.
Micah's life inspires his friends, family
By Jill Rothenberg

Like many other kids his age, Belleview School seventh grader Micah Chase loves to play basketball, improve his Nintendo game and hang out with friends. And although Micah, 13, was diagnoses last June with myelodysplastic syndrome, a form of leukemia, he won't let it slow him down.

"He's never let his illness be a factor in anything he does, whether it's his behavior in class or his work on the basketball court," said Pete Larkin, Micah's teacher and basketball coach. "He's my point guard," he said. "Even if he's running out of gas, he still wants to go out and play."

Amid the shouts of the fans and calls of the cheerleaders, Micah joined his team last night in their game against Don Pedro Elementary. "He puts all his heart and soul into it," said his mother, Shelley, as Micah dribbled down the court and fired a pass at a teammate.

Micah spent time at Oakland Children's Hospital last summer, where he became good friends with his nurse, Debbie Atencio. "He's funny, smart, and mature beyond his years," Atencio said. "We talked about some tough times and he always has a great ability to understand what's going on."

Micah has made an effort to understand his illness, but he doesn't let it interrupt his life," added his father, Del. "He's been real aggressive about asking questions," his dad said. "He knows what's going on, understands the lingo, and he knows that no one can watch out for him as well as he can."

Friends are important to Micah. "I like playing with all my friends," he said as he gathered around the television with his cousins, Levi and Season Zukal, and his brother Nick, who were playing video games.

With his cousins, his brother, and his dogs, Butchy and Pepper, Micah relaxed in his family's cozy living room after the basketball game. Asked about his favorite subject in school, he said, "recess," as a smile crossed his face.

Micah is a 49er and Giants fan and particularly enjoys football, which he hasn't been able to play since he got ill. And like millions of other football fans, he will be watching his favorite sport on television this Sunday.

"I want the Redskins to win," he said.

"Micah's courage has been inspirational to everyone around him," said his aunt, Jan Zukal. "He's been so phenomenal through the whole thing," she said. "He's gone through more in the last six months than we'll go through in our lives."

Micah has not let his illness change his life, said family friend Terry Gonzales. "He just wants to be a regular Joe," she said. "He could be sitting around feeling sorry for himself, but that's not what he chooses to do. I'm so proud of him and he's not even my own child."

"He stays real active," said another family friend, Patti Young. "I think that's what gives him the energy to keep going."

Micah's pediatrician in Sonora, Kelly George, also finds Micah's energy and positive attitude inspiring. "Micah's always been very upbeat," he said. "He's shown a tremendous amount of courage and inner strength."

Two community events will be held to help Micah and others with leukemia find bone marrow donors. A spaghetti dinner and auction will be held Sunday, February 2nd at the Elks Lodge in Sonora to raise money for the donor drive on February 15th.

--used with permission of
The Union Democrat

Chapter 7

It is a beautiful drive through the heart of Central California and up into the foothills of the Sierra Nevada. Tiny creeks cut through the rolling hills here and there, recognized only by a glitter of sunlight, a sudden dab of green in a pallet mostly brown. Wildflowers populate the hills in spring -- purple lupine, orange poppies, blue brodiaeas. Remnants of history left by the Chinese immigrants mark the persistence of their hard working hands in the faces of stone fences, still holding on with the passage of time. Tombstone slate stands erect and true to its name, populating the hills, creating the illusion of small cemeteries. My parents often took my sisters and me on Sunday drives to Sonora and to Columbia. Those trips marked the beginning of my love for the area. When I first moved to Sonora in the mid 1970's, addresses outside the city limit were still rural routes. The first stop light in Tuolumne County was yet to be installed. I had a great infatuation with the high country granite, the lakes and rivers, the pines and cedars. I also loved the local history. Sonora is in the heart of 49er country; fortunes were made here during the California Gold Rush era. What I quickly grew to realize, however, was that the greatest wealth of the county was the people themselves. Most came here for the

74

peace and quiet, the rural atmosphere, the love of space and community pride. In the majority of cases, neighbors are friends and strangers are treated with respect. Over the years, it has never ceased to amaze me how the community comes together in times of need, how busy people find the time to help at a fundraiser -- organizing, collecting donations, cooking food, playing music. Others, with little in their pockets, dig a little deeper to help someone less fortunate.

This community outpouring of support held true for Micah. Friends gathered items from local merchants for the auction that was to be held at his benefit: gift baskets, baseball memorabilia, paintings by local artists, ski lift tickets, vouchers for overnight lodging, dinners for two at nearby restaurants. Local professionals and artisans offered their services: dental exams and cleanings, tree pruning services, free road gravel, firewood, custom-made golf clubs and a handmade fly fishing rod.

"People come in to our store and say, 'Here. Here's twenty bucks. Just people off the street who see the benefit flier in the window, the picture with that kid smiling," said family friends, Craig and Roseanne Gottlieb, who owned a local coin shop. *"He's an All-American kid,"* we tell folks who ask. *"He's bright-eyed, he plays sports, he's involved with other kids, he's a good student. He's all you imagine when you say All-American kid."*

The Sonora Elks Club offered their building, and various markets supplied the ingredients for a spaghetti dinner. On the night of Micah's fundraiser, people from the Elks Lodge prepared and cooked the food. Micah's friends, his brother Nick, cousins Kip, Katy, Levi, and Season, served plates heaping with spaghetti and cleared the

75

tables when people were finished eating.

The outpouring of love, the generosity of everyone involved, was overwhelming. Amid a backdrop of live country-rock music, Micah visited with friends and supporters there to help him raise money to find a cure. More than 650 people came to the Elks Lodge raising $11,000.00 to be matched dollar-for-dollar by the *Heart of America*, allowing almost four-hundred donors to be tested free-of-charge -- four-hundred new names added to the national bone marrow donor registry. "Surely, one of these people," Micah whispered in my ear, "will be my match." He smiled and kissed my cheek. His eyes scanned the faces of those in the room, ever hopeful as he walked away to mingle with the crowd. One of Micah's friends that night compared his courage and tenacity to that of Magic Johnson. *"He doesn't let his disease get in the way of his living,"* Adam said. *"He knows he has it, but he doesn't sit around and dwell on it. He lives his life to the fullest."* As I watched Micah talk with his friends, laughing, helping shuffle plates of spaghetti, I marveled at his ability to cope.

The search for donors didn't stop in Sonora. My sister Carol was busy organizing three marrow drives in Modesto. Del's sister, Chris, and his mother, Dolores, found people near their homes in northern California -- Los Molinos and Red Bluff -- willing to be tested as a possible match. I made a phone call to the publisher of a Choctaw newspaper in Oklahoma, and an ad was placed, along with a picture of Micah, requesting that people come forward and be tested for a possible match.

In June of 1992, Micah was put on a new kind of medication: 5 azacytadine. This drug was part of a study, but unlike DCTER, the purpose of the regimen was not to cure Micah's leukemia, only to hold his counts in a stable position, buying us time to find a donor. Lab work was done weekly, every Friday, like clockwork. I drew the blood myself, filling tube after tube from Micah's Broviac catheter. We had the routine down to a science; Micah would lie down on the couch and hold the purple-topped tubes after I filled them. I would flush the line, clean the insertion site, re-dress the area with sterile gauze and tape. Nick helped by bringing me extra alcohol pads if I needed them, standing by with Betadine swabs and dressing pads.

Our daily trip to the mailbox produced handfuls of mail. I sorted through hospital bills and our insurances' explanation of benefits, creating assorted stacks, watching for any discrepancies or items left unpaid. Time was made every week to double check itemized statements, watching for items that might have been double billed or billed in error. Checks were made out for co-pays and to cover incidentals related to our trips back and forth to Oakland. So far, we had been lucky. Our insurance had covered all hospital stays and related billings.

Micah was pale, but strong. Once a month, we went to see Dr. Beach at the clinic for a bone marrow aspirate and biopsy. His body reacted to the new medication as Dr. Beach hoped it would, keeping his blood counts at an 'acceptable' level. The doctors in Sonora collaborated with the doctors in Oakland. Following the specifications and parameters set by Oakland Children's, Sonora Community Hospital agreed to treat Micah should he need a transfusion of red blood cells or platelets. Doing that locally rather than going all the way to Oakland saved a day in Micah's life and left him closer to home. *Heart of America* checked the registry every couple of days, watching the numbers for Micah's perfect match.

In Modesto, Carol visited local churches and businesses, passed out flyers, made phone calls, contacted the newspaper and local radio stations to see if they were willing to broadcast the times, dates, and locations for the bone marrow drives she had planned. My sisters and I grew up in Modesto, and we hoped for a strong response. At each drive, people showed up in record numbers -- some we had known since elementary school, junior high or high school -- others we had never met, but were willing to be tested as a possible donor match for Micah. The drives at Doctor's Medical Center and Stanislaus Medical Center were highly successful: the bone marrow drive at Memorial Hospital was the largest single family drive ever held in the state of California and Memorial Hospital matched funds with Heart of America for each person tested. Five hundred and forty-four people were tested that day, and each of them was added to the National Registry for bone marrow donation. My family came away from this massive effort with an enormous sense of awe -- not only was there a ray of hope by way of a potential donor for Micah, but the same could be said of anyone world-wide in need of a *gift of life* through marrow donation.

With the stress mounting, and still no donor match, we decided we needed a break. Every year since my boys were little, we had taken a summer trip to Pacific Grove and Monterey, sometimes to Santa Cruz or Capitola, on occasion to Morro Bay, Pismo Beach, Bodega Bay, Point

Reyes. The summer of 1992 was no different; both boys were asking to go to the ocean, needing a familiar routine, an outing where they could forget about hospitals and blood draws for a couple of days. I packed a special suitcase filled with Micah's Broviac supplies, but other than that, as a family, we were determined to leave his illness behind. We stayed three days at the Lighthouse Lodge in Pacific Grove, playing in the tide pools, in the surf on Asilomar Beach. The coolness of the water, the way it caressed our feet, flowing over, around, and under as we walked, was exhilarating for all of us. Going barefoot was a luxury for Micah these days. A healthy dose of nature was overdue. In the hospital, the nurses told him to wear slip on socks. Even at home, around the house, and out in the yard, he had to have something on his feet. "Too many bugs," Grandma Nellie would say, and she did not mean the crawly kind; germs and viruses were the enemy, and no one ever let Micah forget it.

One morning we drove on the Seventeen Mile Drive along the coast to Carmel. The mountainous slope of white sand that led down to the beach, the water, the roar of the surf, was more than Micah could tolerate. He made the decision to take his shoes off without asking permission, and once he had, there was no turning back. He and Nick stood side-by-side along the shoreline, projecting the same satisfaction as when they built their igloo, working as a team. Both boys left their t-shirts on, running and playing in the ebb of each wave, collected shells and rocks, ignoring but not forgetting the vulnerability of Micah's situation. It was not hard to notice, however, that they avoided a favorite pass time -- building sandcastles, burying each other up to their necks in the warm, white sand. It went unsaid between them, that getting sand in Micah's Broviac could have serious consequences. This was not a suggestion that came from Del or me; it was a decision they made as brothers, without even voicing their concerns.

Later that afternoon we visited Carmel Mission, walked through the courtyard, the gardens, brushing our hands along the old adobe walls, enjoying the smells, the textures, the embedded spirituality. In the chapel, we lit candles, closed our eyes, and prayed. As I finished, I looked up and saw Micah with his hands clasped together, his eyes shut tight, his lips passing an urgent plea to God. Nick and Del placed their candles in a long metal rack beside dozens of others, sending a flock of billowy shadows up the walls, across the pulpit, onto the tomb of Father Junipero Serra. Tears rolled down my cheeks, and for the millionth time, I asked God to heal my little boy; I asked that He grant us enough time to find a donor.

Chapter 8

Our haven that summer was at Grandpa Don's and Grandma Nikki's house in Minden, Nevada. We went as often as we could and whenever Micah was able. It was a place we could relax, where the kids could go boating in the lake behind the house, catch bullfrogs, feed the Mallard Ducks and Canada Geese that wandered over the hilly, quarter-acre lawn. Grandma Nikki spoiled us with her good cooking, and Micah ate with no regard for chemotherapy related stomach problems. He and Nick played with their younger cousins, Oliver and Stewart, sharing their music and teaching them to dance, just laughing, and being boys. Though erring on the side of caution, mischief, as always, was a part of the norm that summer, and the boys looked forward to Grandpa Don's *toys*. On one particular visit, Grandpa bought a shiny green Toro riding lawnmower to replace the old clunker the kids had learned to drive. "Give 'er a test drive," he said, tossing Micah the keys.

The sparkle in Micah's eye and the miniature grin at the corner of his mouth made my stomach flutter. He climbed on the mower, turned the key, and started the engine, disappearing around the far side of the house with Nick running alongside. I stood on the grass, waiting, watching. Minutes passed before I heard their laughter, saw them whip around the side of the house, Micah driving, and Nick seated behind him on the mower. Smiles consumed their faces as they banked the corner, nearly landing themselves and the mower in the lake. As I waved my arms, they slowed to a stop, ready for a safety lecture, a little *time-out.* When they walked into the kitchen to apologize to Grandma Nikki, she had a plate of homemade cookies and two glasses of cold milk waiting on the table, loving them in spite of their shenanigans.

By the fall of that year, Micah was ready for eighth grade. It would mean hard work and difficult choices, balancing homework and hospital, socialization and isolation when his counts were low. He resigned himself early on that there would be no contact sports -- no more wrestling, no baseball, and no basketball. He was getting thinner, and his features were gaunt. There was a noticeable change about his eyes: the spark was missing, the mischievous gleam that was so much a part of Micah's personality had faded. He didn't smile as much. He rarely laughed. I saw him staring at his friends, his cousin Kip, noticing that they were getting taller, maturing into teenagers while he remained in limbo, slowly poisoned by the medicine that was supposed to cure his disease.

Time was the one thing chemotherapy could not hold back. In mid-January of 1993, on the morning of his fourteenth birthday, I took Micah on a shopping spree. He had dropped nearly twenty pounds, and his clothes no longer fit. On the way to town, we went to the hospital lab and dropped off his blood work. We found a barber, one with a sense of humor, someone who would laugh with

Micah while reshaping what there was of his hair. It was important to find the right person; Micah wanted no screw-ups. This was a big day. One he wanted to remember positively. His friends had planned another party, a huge blowout with live music and dancing. There would be no anxious glares, no sympathetic stares. Not today. Not on his birthday.

For the remainder of the afternoon, Micah went about getting ready, proud of his new shirt and pants, happy with his haircut. The phone call came about an hour before he was due to leave for the party. "We're noticing some changes," Dr. Beach said. "Micah's counts are dropping, Shelley. There are blasts showing in his peripheral blood work. He'll need to come in to the hospital."

"He's been doing so well. There must be a mistake." I knew what blasts were -- abnormal cells, leukemia cells. The doctors had seen them in Micah's marrow but never in his circulating blood before.

"You can't make me go, not now!" Micah protested. "Just one party, please, Mom. Just this one!"

"Micah, you can't go. Your counts are too low. You know as well as I do, it's not safe."

"What is safe for me anymore, Mom? Tell me that, will you? I have to live my life, you know. You can't take it all away. Please, please let me go. I'll be good. I won't do anything silly, I promise. I'll go to the hospital right after the party, honest!"

I looked at my son. My heart beat so rapidly, I felt as if it would break free of my chest at any moment. My thoughts bounced from one to the next, none of them providing anything close to a viable solution. If I let him go, he could become dangerously ill, and if I didn't, he might miss a chance that may not come again. Then I, not he, would regret it for the rest of my life. I packed Micah's suitcase and waited, sweating through three long hours while Micah had the time of his life.

When we got to Oakland Children's, nothing much had changed. Dr. Feusner was there, but not nearly as visible as he had been on our previous visits. Dr. Beach worked in the clinic, not on the fifth floor, and although she could sneak a visit now and again, she was not Micah's primary physician when he was admitted into the hospital. Micah grimaced when *Dr. Doom* walked into the room. She rarely brought good news, and the look on her face most often suggested something neither of us wanted to hear. The plan was to administer a new type of chemotherapy. This protocol was short but aggressive.

In the week prior to coming to the hospital, Micah complained several times about pains in his legs. At the hospital, after Micah's course of chemotherapy, the pains became excruciating. He shook uncontrollably, moaning when I tried to move him or if he had to stand up for any reason. He developed large areas of rash that looked like bruises. Specialists were called in. Doctor after doctor took tests, asked for x-rays, biopsies. One doctor said the symptoms presented like osteonecrosis, a disease resulting from the temporary or permanent loss of the blood supply to the bones. "Without blood," he explained, "the bone tissue dies and causes the bone to collapse. Necrosis often affects long bones such as the femur, the bone extending from the knee to the hip, as is the case with Micah."

Exacerbated by the corticosteroids Micah had been

84

taking, the symptoms of necrosis had progressed to an unbearable level. The rash was diagnosed as *erythema nodosum*, an inflammation of the fat cells under the skin. "It's the worst case we've ever seen in a child," the doctor said. "With your permission, we'd like to take some pictures. There's a woman in San Francisco who's writing a textbook on rashes, and she would like to include Micah as a case for study."

"Great," Micah said, trying to smile. "Again I'm the one with the worst/best scenario?"

The nurses followed the only suggested course of treatment. They elevated Micah's legs and applied cool wet cloths to make him more comfortable, hoping the symptoms would subside over time. A few days later Micah developed a fungal infection and was given Amphotericin again. Within hours of administration, he was shivering so violently that no heated blanket, no amount of Benadryl could calm him down. Once more, I lay next to him on the bed, trying to warm him with my body while his teeth chattered and tears rolled down his cheeks.

Upon his release, Micah was provided with a walker, but he refused to use it once we exited the hospital. He limped to the parking garage, lips set, fists clinched, determined to get to the car on his own. I felt his frustration and understood his need to be free of hospital devices. Both he and I had had enough this trip and were ready to go home.

In February, we took a family vacation to Hawaii. It was Micah's dream to visit the beaches there, and since his condition had stabilized, Dr. Beach encouraged us to go while we could. Grandma Nellie made the trip possible, buying airfare for everyone, including aunts, uncles, and cousins. Auntie Carol and Uncle Kip arranged for motel rooms through a co-op at their business, planning all the details of the trip. We had Micah's Broviac catheter removed before we left, so he could swim without worry, keep up with Nick, and his cousins. For the first week, we stayed in the King Kamehameha Kona Beach Hotel on the big island of Hawaii. The hotel had a private beach in a cove surrounded by palm trees. An immaculately kept lawn swept curvaceously around the sand, leading to a small marina and Kailua Bay. We watched the busy boat rental shop -- people with pleasure boats, waverunners, and catamarans heading out into the bay beyond the hotel cove, traversing, circling, churning up white caps on a calm blue sea while we swam, snorkeled and soaked up the sun. The ambiance of the Kona Coast, the aura and tranquility around the town of Kailua made it easy for us to relax, to forget for moments at a time, the reason we were there. The kids explored on their own a bit, down the sidewalks through town, through the surf shops and sandwich shacks close to the hotel. We rented two cars and explored the island, snorkeling with sea turtles at Kahaluu Beach, walking along the black sand at Punaluu Beach, trekking the path to Akaka Falls. We visited Parker Ranch, Hilo, and Mount Kilauea.

Even within our moments of peace, the reality of Micah's illness was ever-present in the shadows. As smoke belched from the heart of Mount Kilauea, I saw Micah's cousins, Season and Katy, off on their own, standing with their heads down, their hands clasped together. In front of them, on the edge of the volcano were offerings of bananas

86

and oranges, coconuts, and flowers. Katy was ten years old, and Season only seven -- but still they understood that those offerings were a part of a prayer. Season held a few wildflowers she had picked along the road somewhere, and together, she and Katy added the flowers to the shrine. Again, they stood in silence, praying for Micah, I knew. Micah walked up to the girls and took hold of Season's hand. He leaned down and put a feather he had found beside the fruit and flowers. Nick, Kip, and Levi joined them, pulling pink puka shells, brown and white spotted cowry shells from their pockets, setting them carefully beside the rest. Grandma Nellie, aunties and uncles, Del and I watched, feeling amazed at and proud of the children we had raised.

Slack key guitar music, lanais, hot tubs, and luaus filled our evenings. On our last night on the Big Island, we watched the sky turn gold at sunset, saw it yawn and stretch along the horizon, as Micah and Kip, Nick and Katy, Levi and Season, played football on the sand at Hapuna Beach State Park. The thought of leaving paradise brought tears to my eyes. I wanted a magic wand. I wanted a machine to stop time. A spell cast. A prayer answered. I wanted a camera to capture Micah in that instant, on the beach, running and jumping for the football, silhouetted in perfection, with the ocean he loved as a backdrop. I wanted to rewind the clock, to stop whatever it was that I had done, or not done, to cause the leukemia to strike him in the first place. I wanted it gone. I wanted to stay in Hawaii with my boys, healthy and whole, forever. I would have promised anything, given up everything, our house, possessions, my job. If only.

We spent the following week in Honolulu, on Oahu, staying at the Outrigger on Waikiki Beach. The kids learned to surf and explored the International Marketplace; we took a ride on a catamaran, watched surfing contests at the Pipeline, visited the Waimea State Park. We climbed to the top of Diamondhead, went to a hula show, laughing while Grandma Nellie did the hula with a King Kamehameha look-alike. For seven more days, we forgot about Oakland Children's Hospital. We left blood draws and platelet counts and biopsies in California while we played and ate and swam through Micah's dream vacation. He never slowed down. The only clues suggestive of his illness were his occasional limp and the blotchy sunburn surrounding the catheter scar on his chest.

The airplane ride from Honolulu to San Francisco was long and tiring. As we stepped out of the baggage claim area at the end of our flight, we saw a huge white limousine parked at the curb in front of the Hawaiian Airlines terminal. A chauffer held up a sign with Micah's name written on it. Uncle Kip had arranged for a friend of theirs to drive the kids from San Francisco to Modesto, in style. "Cool!" Micah said. "What an amazing end to a perfect trip."

The kids piled into the limo with Grandma Nellie, and suddenly they were gone. They drove off into the night without me, or Del, or aunties, or uncles. I felt a moment of panic. The magic was gone and suddenly I was terrified. There was no balance, no peace. There was no slack key guitar music to calm me, no sea breeze to pacify my fears. As Del drove, I kept an eye on the car carrying both of our children, trying to focus on the excitement they must feel

88

while riding with their cousins in a limo for the first time, rather than the anxiousness in my belly. Passing through Oakland on the way home, I saw the eternal lights of the Children's Hospital in the distance, closed my eyes, and imagined them as tiki torches, casting shadows over the sand on Hapuna Beach.

Chapter 9

When the doctors removed Micah's Broviac prior to our trip to Hawaii, they inserted a port-a-cath in its place. The device was about the size of a quarter and had been placed under Micah's skin between his breast and shoulder bones. There were no tubes and there was no external access, thus his freedom to swim at will. Should he have needed a transfusion or any other medication, the device could have been accessed by a single poke.

Upon returning from our trip, Micah was prescribed low-dose chemotherapy. He wore an automatic pump clipped to his pants, which fed a regulated dose of his medication through tubing into the port-a-cath. Micah monitored his medications as well as I did at that point, keeping his own record of blood draws, and the blood counts that came after.

The phone call I had been dreading came one afternoon, early in June. "Micah's last test results weren't good," Dr. Beach told me. "It's time to discuss transplant options at UCSF with Dr. Calloway again. I can schedule an appointment at your earliest convenience."

I phoned my sister Carol after speaking to Dr. Beach. "She wants us to talk with the transplant team in San Francisco, but she's checking into alternatives as well. She asked if we'd be willing to fly overseas to Italy, maybe, or Germany. Anywhere, I told her, just tell us where to go and we'll get Micah there. She also spoke with a doctor in Texas. They're performing half-match bone marrow transplants at a hospital there, with promising results."

"Okay, what do we do?" Carol asked.

"We're going to San Francisco on Friday to meet with Dr. Calloway," I told her.

"All of you?"

"Yes. Dr. Calloway wants to meet with Micah. We'll go to UCSF and later to Pier 39, so the boys can have a little fun."

Del, Micah, Nick and I left early Friday morning, stopping for breakfast in Manteca, passing through Oakland, crossing the Bay Bridge by 8:30 a.m. Micah's appointment with Dr. Calloway was at 9:30. We arrived at the University Hospital and found our way to the transplant unit, exploring a little, taking our time. Micah and Nick wandered in the hallway near the waiting room, checking things out, but staying within earshot. The canvas travel bag I stocked specifically for road trips, filled with paper and colored pencils, crossword puzzles, books, peanuts, fruit snacks, and granola bars was of no interest to either of them. They were nervous, fidgeting, talking quietly to each other. When a nurse took us into an examining room, Nick sat on my lap. Micah sat in a chair beside me, preparing for the usual routine by baring his forearm for a blood pressure check. It reminded me of times at Oakland Children's Hospital when he would raise his little arm automatically as the room light went on in the middle of the night. Half asleep, he would submit to examinations, even needle

91

pokes, by rote and without a complaint. Feeling stunned by how easily this had happened, how we had adapted as a family to life after leukemia, I felt a great need to hug them all, and hold them tight. Del was standing by the doorway, pretending not to be nervous, giving the equipment in the room a once over, as had become his habit. Nick held my hand, looking away as the nurse checked Micah's eyes, ears, and throat. I squeezed him a little tighter.

When Dr. Calloway came in, Micah stood up and shook his hand. "I'm so glad to meet you," Dr. Calloway told him. "You're a star patient according to the doctors at Oakland Children's." Dr. Calloway did a quick examination, listening to Micah's heartbeat, his lung sounds. "Do you understand why you're here today?" he asked.

"Yes," Micah said. "I'm here to find out about having a bone marrow transplant."

"Do you know why you need to have a transplant?"

"Yes. I know."

"It's not going to be easy."

"I know, but I don't care. I'm strong. I want to have a transplant. I know it's my only chance, and I want to live." Micah looked straight at Dr. Calloway. There was no hesitation in his eyes, only a display of his spirit, his commitment to fight the odds.

Dr. Calloway stared back at him, obviously touched. "Micah, we're going to do what we can, I promise you that. Right now, I need to talk with your parents for a bit. My nurse will get you and your brother some juice and cookies. There's a waiting room with a television set just across the hall. You can wait there."

Micah was hesitant, not used to being excluded from

any conversation regarding his care. I went with him and Nick to the waiting room, reassured them, and got them settled and then returned to Del and Dr. Calloway in the examining room. As Dr. Calloway explained it, the only option for Micah at UCSF was a T-cell depleted transplant. There was only a ten percent chance that Micah would survive that type of transplant and a seventy percent chance the leukemia would return after. He described the reason for such a large relapse factor: "Some graft versus host is necessary to attack any blast cells that might be left following the transplant. In a T-cell depleted transplant, all T-cells, a type of lymphocyte, are destroyed, thus eliminating any chance of GVH. With the type of leukemia Micah has, we feel that some GVH is necessary to assure a permanent remission. We've consulted with specialists in Los Angeles and in New York, and they concur with our opinion. A T-cell depleted transplant is *not* the optimal treatment in Micah's case. That said, if this remains his only choice, we *will* offer Micah the transplant. Please," he said, "make no mistake, we want to help Micah any way we can. I wish I had better news."

Before we left, Dr. Calloway assured us again that he would hold a bed space for Micah at the transplant unit. Since our insurance company had already preauthorized payment for a bone marrow transplant, he anticipated no problems there. He said he would discuss the situation with Dr. Beach and Dr. Feusner, making sure they were apprised of his offer to transplant Micah, should we choose to go that route.

By the next afternoon, Dr. Beach had phoned Ketchell Hospital in Texas to discuss Micah's options with their transplant specialist. She called me right afterward: "I'm very excited about this," she said. "Having reviewed Micah's treatment history and knowing his current condition, Dr. Allen feels that the transplant they're offering at Ketchell is his best chance for a cure. They're saying it's at 45%, Shelley. That's really good, considering the odds at UCSF. Micah's blast count is rising," Dr. Beach continued. "The drug we're using to hold his counts is no longer working. Continuing cycles of chemotherapy might buy us a small window of time, but those treatments will be tough on him, so we want to avoid that route if we can. We want to keep him as strong as possible for transplant."

"So you think Texas is our best option?" I asked.

"Yes," she said. "I do. I'll speak with you more about it at Micah's clinic visit next week."

A smile crossed Micah's face. His eyes lit up. "My life, my decision?" he asked.

Both Dr. Beach and I nodded our heads. "Yes, Micah," I said. "Your body, your choice."

"Then yes, I want to do it. I want to go for it."

"You're a fighter, Micah, the best I've ever seen," Dr. Beach told him.

Micah talked all the way home, was more animated than I had seen him since Hawaii. He told Del about the transplant in Texas and that he had decided he wanted to go for it. Del agreed, as I had, that we should move forward as quickly as possible. Micah and Nick helped with dinner, did their homework, and later, we finished reading the last chapter of the *Fellowship of the Ring*. After tucking them into bed, I went back into the living room and turned on the television. Jane Seymour's character, Dr. Mike, on _Dr. Quinn, Medicine Woman,_ was performing surgery on her adopted son Brian. He had fallen out of a tree while pretending to be an eagle, lost his sight, and lapsed into a coma. I couldn't help wonder what she would do in my situation, when the odds were at a mere 45%.

As the television program progressed, Dr. Mike did everything she could to save her son. Even with her primitive instruments and sterilization procedures that were minimal at best, she fought the odds. Like Micah, Brian loved eagles, and he loved climbing trees. He was a bit too daring, and he was strong-willed. Like me, Dr. Mike would do anything, go anywhere, risk everything to save her child. Suddenly the 60% chance of survival I had panicked over during Micah's first stay at Oakland Children's Hospital seemed tame and left me wishing for just that; a 60% chance would seem like a miracle at this point. As the thought took hold, everything around me blurred, including the television screen, Dr. Mike and her son Brian. If left up to me in that instant the boy would have come out of the surgery permanently blinded. My hands were shaking, my chest convulsing slightly in the aftermath of a sudden burst of tears. I prayed that I could do better, handle things better when it came to the final test of courage, for me, for Micah, for Del, and for Nick.

The protocol for the procedure at Ketchell Hospital called for the use of various immunosuppressants, including Interleukin-2 to reduce the risk of graft versus host disease. 'Reduce' being the optimal word. The results of the HLA typing Del and I had participated in early in Micah's treatment showed that Del was the best choice for a half-match transplant; therefore, he would be Micah's donor. Under light anesthesia, the doctors at Ketchell would extract some marrow cells from Del's hipbone. He would be groggy for awhile and sore for a few days afterward, but that was it. After the transplant, Micah would be in isolation, and then he would need time to recuperate, preferably close to the hospital. We could be gone for several months, maybe up to a year. I wondered how I could manage and what would be best for Micah and for Nick. For two years, our family had been apart as much as we had been together. Being away from Nick for any length of time was unacceptable, and having him with us would be a huge factor in Micah's recuperation. Nick needed to be a part of that healing time, for his own well-being as well as for Micah's. And I needed both of them; if I were going to be strong for Micah, I needed Nick close by. That much was a given.

The administrators at Belleview School, the school board, and faculty granted me all the time I needed. Del would be able to take leave from his mechanics job with the County, but there were financial concerns at stake; we had no reserves to pull on as far as savings or other viable securities. We could sell our house, but that would be a last resort. We decided that Del, Micah, and I would make the trip initially, leaving Nick with my sister Jan and her family and with Grandma Nellie. Del would fly home after the transplant, keeping Nick on as normal a schedule as was possible, traveling to Houston whenever possible. As soon as Micah was released from the hospital and we were settled in a house, Nick would come to stay, possibly starting school there in the fall. Del and I would make a decision about short or long term residence, depending on Micah's stability and recuperation status.

I talked with my mother and both my sisters, securing plans for Nick, setting up a schedule for house sitting while we were gone. Our neighbors, Terry and Denise, Chris and Caitie, agreed to feed the animals and water the plants. The logistics of where we would stay when we got to Houston, details about the transplant, the hospital, were still vague. "Do you have a date set?" my sister Carol asked. "Has the paperwork been submitted, both to Ketchell Hospital, and the insurance company?"

"Dr. Beach is working on that now. A bone marrow transplant was pre-approved by the insurance company for San Francisco, so we don't anticipate any problems."

"What about the donor drives? No word about a possible match?"

"No. And we can't wait any longer. The sooner we get this done, the better chance we have for a cure. Micah is getting worse, Carol. I can feel it. If you look past his smile into his eyes, there's such sadness; it's as if he's only half here, and that scares me to death.

"The doctors say this type of transplant has a great potential for success. There's a man at Ketchell who's had this same procedure. He is four months out of isolation and doing really well. Another person, a woman, is still in isolation, but so far her counts show a remission. Micah will be the youngest to receive this protocol, but they've given his age and need great consideration." "

"And Micah?"

"He wants to go for it. You should have seen him when Dr. Beach told us about this transplant. He's so

97

careful with himself right now, doing everything he can to stay healthy. Dr. Beach's been in constant contact with the doctors at Ketchell Hospital, reporting changes, monitoring Micah's condition. The doctors in Oakland and in Houston agree that Micah is a good candidate. He could get through this and go into remission."

"Okay, then," Carol said. "Let's do this."

On June 16th, I got a phone call from hospital admissions coordinator at Ketchell Hospital asking for Micah's social security number, and birth date. On June 22nd, I spoke with them again, verifying my birth date, insurance information, verification of employment. I phoned the hospital's business office later that day to discuss any possible concerns. "Micah will be a direct admit," the clerk told me. "The patient is pre-certified. I see no problems."

Ketchell Hospital gave the go ahead. The transplant was scheduled for June 29th, a week after Micah's eighth grade graduation ceremony. He would miss the dance and his class trip to Marriott's Great America, but he would be able to attend the graduation itself if all went well. He had written a speech and planned to give it. There would be no telling him otherwise.

When Micah was a toddler, he would climb over any barricade I put in his way. No matter how tall or wide, he would maneuver his arms and legs until he hoisted himself over the top, on his way to whatever adventure had attracted his attention. One winter when he was nine and Nick was seven, they decided to go for a walk in the snow. Micah insisted he was responsible enough to get his brother and himself back safely, that he had a good sense of direction, and could find his way home. An hour later, I was trudging through the snow, calling their names, feeling slightly panicked by the time I heard their screams of laughter. Having made a homemade toboggan out of an old piece of wood, they were careening down a steep slope, through a thick grove of pine trees, past boulders, and toward a ditch full of water. Wet but happy, they succumbed to a scolding as they climbed back up the hill, racing home to a warm bath, a cup of hot chocolate, and at story time a modern version of Red-Riding Hood, about two little boys, traveling unprotected in the woods.

As they grew older, my boys tried to wean me of being so protective. They took bicycle rides down the steep, curving back roads from our house into Columbia. They played with garter snakes on sticks -- too close in resemblance to a rattlesnake to suit my comfort level. I dealt with skinned knees, battered elbows, and black eyes. None of that, however, prepared me for the nightmare we were facing.

On June 24th, Micah was admitted into Oakland Children's Hospital as a precautionary measure. He was started on intravenous antibiotics to prevent any possibility of an infection so close to transplant. His excitement was palpable. He was alert and full of questions, buzzing with enthusiasm. The following morning, he underwent surgery to have his port-a-cath removed and a second Broviac catheter inserted -- one that could withstand the toxicity of the chemotherapy he would receive during transplant. Later, he talked on the phone with family and friends, sharing his excitement about his upcoming trip to Texas.

99

"I've never been there," he told Grandma Nellie. "Do you think I'll come back wearing a cowboy hat and spurs?"

Del talked with a friend who would take us to the airport in San Francisco. We purchased airline tickets. Thanks to our good friends, and the community of Sonora, a trust fund established in Micah's name would provide the money for travel expenses and short term lodging once we got to Houston.

Dr. Beach came to talk with me on the morning of June 25th. She happened to catch me in the hallway, after a trip to the restroom. "I spoke with Dr. Allen," she said. "A representative from your insurance company phoned Ketchell Hospital yesterday, saying there's a hang-up with the authorization. Dr. Allen apologized. She sounded as shocked as I am. We really didn't anticipate any problems."

"I thought it was all set? We were told Micah was pre-certified." A million tiny prickles raced up and down my spine. My lips felt numb.

"I know," Dr. Beach said. "I can't believe it either. We're going to keep pushing, Shelley. Don't worry. We're going to get Micah to Houston as soon as we can."

I could see Micah watching us through the window, aware of the expression on my face, the sudden shift of Dr. Beach's posture. When I walked back in the room, he was visibly shaken. "What's wrong?" he asked. "Why didn't you talk in here?" His eyes followed mine, searching for the truth.

"Oh, honey, Dr. Beach was on her way to the clinic," I told him. "She just happened to see me in the hallway, that's all." I sat beside him and told him not to worry.

100

"There's a little bit of a hang up. It'll be a few more days before we can go to Houston. Just a few more days, I promise."

Micah's shoulders fell, his chest sank. It was as if his body caved in on itself. "Mom," he pleaded. "Please make this happen. Please, Mom. I know it will work."

Telephone conversations continued between Oakland Children's and Ketchell Hospital. The transplant was officially postponed by the Ketchell transplant specialist due to the insurance company's questions about authorization of payment. Del cancelled our airline tickets and asked our friend if he could stand ready to drive us to the airport at a later date. A doctor from the insurance company phoned Dr. Beach, asking about her reasons for wanting to send Micah to Houston. She explained Micah's situation and the urgency as far as time constraints.

While we waited for an answer, Micah was released and sent home. He cried upon leaving the hospital. It was the first time he'd done that in his two years of treatment. On July 5th Dr. Beach received a fax from Ketchell Hospital stating, "Insurance cleared. Dr. Collier and Dr. Klu will see Micah here in pediatrics to evaluate. Thanks." Once again, we prepared to go to Houston, expecting to leave within the next few days. Micah seemed tentative, but ready.

On July 6th, Ketchell Hospital got a fax from the insurance company asking for a letter of necessity. Ketchell Hospital sent the requested letter immediately, again stating the urgency of Micah's situation:

July 8, 1993
Attention: Medical review
RE: Micah Chase
To Whom It May Concern:

Micah Chase is a fourteen year old patient diagnosed with acute myelocytic leukemia. His disease is in drug resistance relapse at this time. Phase 1 and 2 agents have been ineffective. He recently received Ara-C with a toxic non-response.

This disease is insensitive to chemotherapy. He is unlikely to be cured with conventional dose treatment. The only therapy capable of curing his disease at this stage is bone marrow transplantation.

In order to perform bone marrow transplantation a donor must be identified. HLA typing of family members failed to identify a completely suitable bone marrow donor for this patient. Unrelated histocompatible donors are not available. In this setting, successful transplants have been achieved with haploidentical family donors. The father would be the family member donor for Micah.

The transplant procedure required hospitalization and supportive care for long periods in protective isolation. The patient receives supralathal chemotherapy and whole body radiation to destroy the malignant bone marrow and systemic disease prior to receiving the healthy marrow from the normal donor. Substantial experience with haploidentical transplants have been reported over the last decade. Progress in the management of graft-related toxicities has improved the outlook and outcome substantially.

As indicated by the attached letters from the National Institutes of Health, this is not an experimental form of therapy. This is a

102

documented, effective form of therapy and the best available treatment in this setting. We and other bone marrow transplant centers are continuing clinical research with the goal of further improving the results.

Due to the unstable medical condition of this patient, it is urgent that we proceed quickly with the bone marrow transplantation of the healthy marrow. We need confirmation of this patient's insurance coverage for bone marrow transplant costs and marrow procurement from the father. We are requesting a written, clearly worded confirmation within one week of this application.

Sincerely,
Dr. Albert Collier
Bone Marrow Transplantation Service

On the 8th of July, Dr. Bustoff from the insurance company faxed Ketchell Hospital, stating that a final decision was not possible until he received a "precise protocol which applied to this child" and asking for data characterizing the success of this treatment for Micah's condition.

The protocol abstract and informed consent which would be used for Micah was faxed to Dr. Bustoff by Ketchell Hospital, as requested, on July 9th. Also on July 9th, Dr. Beach received a call from Ketchell Hospital. "There's been a mistake," the patient relations representative told her. "The only clearance we have from the insurance company is for a clinic visit. I'm sorry for the confusion."

Chapter 10

According to our latest confirmed plans, we had been re-scheduled to be in Houston to start transplant preparedness on July 12th. There was no point in going if the insurance clearance was only for a clinic visit. The look Micah gave me when I told him was one a mother never wants to face. I felt like a liar. I felt as if I had deceived him all these years with my preaching about the rightness of the world, about peace, and love, and understanding. All that I had taught him about the basic goodness of people, a belief in fair and just outcomes for those who work hard enough was desecrated by the disbelief I saw in his eyes, the total and justifiable fear.

He began questioning other aspects of his medical bills, whether they had been covered by insurance in the past. He watched for their arrival in the mail, and I found him searching through envelopes occasionally, perusing the blue insurance explanation of benefit forms, unsure what he was looking for, but still needing to see. Del and I tried to assure him that all was well, but he was too astute not to realize a change in the type of groceries we bought, the extras we no longer purchased.

Confounded by Micah's disappointment and fear was my knowledge that his blast count was rising. His condition otherwise was stable, but any change in that stability could cause a diminished chance of success after transplant. In other words, another delay would be extremely detrimental. Along with his rising blast count, there was a constant worry that he might develop an infection, spike a fever. His platelet count and his red-cell count were also matters of concern. Transfusions can cause undue stress and the added possibility of complications, such as another fungal infection. Micah's doctors concurred that the best course of treatment at that point was as little treatment as possible. He would continue to have weekly blood draws and transfusions if necessary, but that was it; they wanted to keep his body as free of chemicals and chemotherapy related agents as possible. Dr. Beach, acting as spokesperson for Micah's team of doctors at Oakland and in San Francisco, stressed the fact that Micah needed to get to Houston *now*, to have his transplant *now*, while his body was still strong enough to withstand the rigors of the treatment. Why wasn't anyone listening to her? A day could bring dramatic change to a child in Micah's condition. A week could alter his world. Two weeks could mean the difference between of life or death. Why the insurance company could not see that was beyond my understanding. I felt like tearing my hair out at the roots, screaming at the top of my lungs to make sure somebody heard my frustration.

On July 14th, I received a call from Ketchell Hospital's financial coordinator. "Mrs. Chase, I'm afraid there's a problem."

"What's new," I felt like saying, but held my tongue.

"Your insurance company is refusing to pay for the

105

transplant. We have their official denial of payment."

"What? That can't be! We've sent them everything they need! This can't be happening!"

"I know, I'm sorry. They say they never cleared 'this' type of transplant. They say it's considered experimental."

"Every protocol Micah has been on has been considered experimental! I've got every study protocol right here in front of me." I read the titles of each: "Study CCG 2891. Study CCG 0926. Study for the efficacy of 5-Azacytidine in Myelodysplastic Syndrome. What about those? Studies, every one! And the insurance company never complained about paying for those treatment protocols and their associated hospital stays!"

"I know. I'm so sorry."

"Please, can you fax me a copy of their letter?"

July 14, 1993

To: Sally Roads
Patient Relations Representative
Ketchell Hospital

Re: Micah Chase

We have reconsidered the request for benefits for the haploidentical BMT for Micah Chase, who has drug resistant acute leukemia. The reconsideration included discussion with several independent academic hands-on bone marrow transplant hematologists, as well as a discussion with Dr. Collier at Ketchell Hospital.

Based on this reconsideration, the denial is upheld. Contrary to the form letter you sent, this is an experimental procedure, as

106

clearly stated in the protocol, which was subsequently sent to me. The insurance company contracts exclude coverage for investigational or experimental procedures. This is an interesting protocol, however, we would expect the care which patients receive in the course of this protocol to be covered by research grants.

Professionally yours,
David Bustoff, MD

Two days later, Micah was back in the hospital spiking a fever of 103 degrees. It came out of nowhere; there were no visible signs of infection. They hit him with massive amounts of antibiotics, keeping in mind his growing need for a transplant. I sat by silently while Tom tried to lift his spirits, but something had changed. The sparkle was missing, the circumstances of life having hit him bluntly on the head. My fear was hard to hide as it became more obvious that no amount of encouragement, nothing I said or did, was helping Micah out of his depression. Finally, at Debbie's suggestion, I left his room, waiting out his refusal to take any medication, seeking solace in my journal:

"Micah is becoming stubborn about taking his pills, and he refuses to do his mouth care. I am worn out, my patience is thin. Each attempt I make to calm him down seems only to make things worse. It's painful to see and worse to imagine the repercussions this behavior could bring about. I'm afraid. I'm so afraid. And so I sit and wait, and it is with all my strength that I stay out in this hallway, listening as Debbie gently reprimands Micah for not taking meds, reminding him how important they are if he wants to heal and go home.

She's doing my job. What's the matter with me?

He's calling me, "Mom! Come back here! Mom, where are you?"

It's all I can do not to give in and go back into his room, to take him in my arms and tell him it's all okay, that he is okay, and that the medications can be set aside for now. I can see Debbie's face, her kind eyes, and I know she's right. I must stay here. I must wait. Here.

Oh, dear God, it's quiet now. Oh, thank God, Micah is taking his pills. He's looking at the door, looking for me. It's over, for now, thank God, it's over.

Later that same day, Dr. Beach requested that I meet her in her office. "Micah's transplant has been postponed until we get this straightened out," she said with regret. "Believe me, we'll fight this, Shelley. The insurance company's denial is simply unacceptable. Micah *will* go to Houston."

"How can they do this?" I asked.

"That's not all," Dr. Beach said. "I've debated whether to tell you this or not, but I feel like I have to. It may do some good and make you angry enough to push harder."

"What?" I asked, hesitantly. In the two years Dr. Beach had been Micah's doctor, I had never seen her so upset.

"I had a conversation with Dr. Bustoff from your insurance company this morning." As Dr. Beach looked at me, I saw her anger, felt her frustration. "Never in my medical career have I been talked to in such a manner," she said. She pushed her chair back and stood up, pacing.

"What did he say," I asked. "Tell me, please." My heart pounded. I stood up.

108

"He told me, 'This kid's going to die anyway. Why should we put that kind of money out'?" Dr. Beach squared off to face me, appalled at the words that just came out of her mouth. "Don't they realize how important this is? Micah needs to go now!" she fumed. "This is unacceptable! I told Dr. Bustoff that Micah wasn't the kind of kid who would accept palliative treatment. It would destroy him to know that there were no other options."

Even though Dr. Beach tried to assure Dr. Bustoff that the proposed bone marrow transplant was not an 'exercise in futility' and that the refusal of Micah's treatment would be medically inappropriate, Dr. Bustoff remained firm about his denial. "The insurance company doctor, getting paid his commission for keeping company expenses down, has made his decision," she told me. "I can't believe that, as Micah's medical doctor, I have less say than he does."

I felt nauseous; dizzy. "This isn't right!" I stammered. "Who is this guy? How can he say something like that? He's putting a price tag on Micah's life! We can't let this happen!"

"As far as I'm concerned, this is a blatant defilement of the medical system," Dr. Beach said. "Something is very wrong when an insurance company has the power to veto a team of practicing physicians, all experts in their field."

At my request, Dr. Beach spoke with Dr. Feusner, Dr. Irwin, and Dr. Calloway, all of whom agreed to fight for Micah's rights. More letters were sent. All the information that was requested by our insurance company was mailed off. One requirement after the other was met, per our insurance company's instructions regarding an appeal.

As the days passed, Micah's depression grew deeper.

He became withdrawn. Dr. Beach took time out of her busy day at the clinic to come and visit. For the first time, in front of her, he cried. "I don't understand," he said. "Are they saying I'm not worth it? Won't they even let me try? I'll do anything, Mom. I'll take my meds. I'll do my mouth care. Please, Dr. Beach, tell them I want to try."

I tried to stay optimistic, to be positive, but it was difficult. My moods matched Micah's minute by minute. We took short walks around the hall. I brought in the video game cart, but even his favorites, Double Dragon and Zelda, barely held his interest. Through an arrangement by a friend, Micah got a phone call from San Francisco 49er, Steve Young. Normally, he would have been ecstatic, but even that was met with meager enthusiasm. He spiked another fever. It came and went in intervals, making us believe that it was a reaction to a medication rather than an infection. The doctors, however, wanted to take no chances and increased his antibiotics, adding new ones, hoping to stabilize him.

"We can't sit by and do nothing," I told Dr. Feusner as I cornered him in the hallway. "We're sending them everything they've asked for. We're doing everything we possibly can." "Make a personal plea, Shelley. I'm not saying it will work," Dr. Feusner said, "but anything is worth a shot at this point."

I wrote a letter, a personal plea for the life of my son, and faxed it directly to Dr. Bustoff at the insurance company:

July 17, 1993
To Whom It May Concern:

I am writing to you regarding your denial of payment for my son Micah's bone marrow transplant. I would like you to please reconsider your decision.

I realize your initial denial was based on the fact that Micah's transplant is by your terms considered experimental. You have a letter signed by Dr. Collier regarding the effectiveness of this treatment, and a letter from the National Institutes of Health, stating that this is not an experimental form of therapy but a documented, effective form under Micah's circumstances. Your letter of denial states that you spoke with Dr. Collier over the phone. Knowing Dr. Collier's commitment to the importance of this type of transplant, his comments couldn't have been anything but supportive of it for Micah.

I have a hard time understanding how, morally or ethically, you can make the judgment to deny payment for Micah's transplant. Most protocols Micah has been on since the beginning of his illness have been or could be considered 'experimental', as could any cancer treatment or transplant of any kind being offered today. The transplant Micah was offered at San Francisco, the T-cell transplant that was pre-approved by you, was considered 'experimental' by your terms. So was the donor match transplant.

Every protocol Micah has been offered, with the exception of his first course of treatment, DCTOR, have been administered to hold his counts until he got a bone marrow transplant. Micah is at a stage in his disease where a decision needed to be made. We realize this transplant is a hard choice, believe me, we have agonized over it ourselves, but it is the only chance for a real cure we have been offered, and Micah desperately wants this chance. We cannot deny him that, and in our eyes, morally, neither can you.

This transplant is Micah's last chance to live. We, as his parents, will do everything we have to do to give him that chance. Because of your hesitancy, and regardless of letters and phone calls from all of Micah's doctors stating the urgency of the situation, we have already lost valuable time.

Please, please reconsider your decision.

Micah's parents,
Shelley and Del Chase

Dr. Beach called me into her office again two days later. "They aren't going for it," she said.

"They can't do that! We'll fight! We'll get a lawyer. What do we do?"

"You do all of that, but first, we need to get Micah his transplant. Ketchell Hospital is asking that you wire them $108,000.00 as a good faith payment. If we can get them the money, Micah can have his clinic visit on July 21st. The transplant will be scheduled for July 23rd."

"My God, I can't believe this. I don't have any money, at least not the kind they're talking about. Does anyone have any decency? Can't they just take him and know we'll fight this thing?"

"Shelley, it all comes down to dollars." Dr. Beach's eyes looked pained. "Sometimes decency flies out the window. You have to know, if it were up to me, I'd get it done, no matter what. Who can you call? Use my phone. Think, Shelley, think."

"Tell them we'll be there. Tell them to hold those dates." Dr. Beach left the room, giving me some privacy. I phoned my mother. By the time she answered, I was barely able to speak.

"Calm down, honey, calm down. Say it all again, slowly this time."

I gulped for air, and began again. "Mom, they won't pay for Micah's transplant, and the hospital in Houston won't admit Micah without money up front."

"Don't panic, just stay by the phone. I'll call you back."

Who, I wondered, will be willing to part with their hard earned money for us, for Micah?

The answer surprised me. My mother, my aunt and my uncle, friends of theirs, friends of ours, all did what they could to raise the $108,000.00 required upfront to admit Micah into the transplant program at Ketchell Hospital. None of them were wealthy. They gathered their savings, dipped into their retirement funds, cashed in annuities to help Micah. My mother was on her own, living on social security and used her nest egg -- most of what she and my father had saved during their lifetime in order to give her grandson a chance at life.

On July 19th, I wired the money to the hospital's financial coordinator via Western Union. On July 20th, we packed our suitcases. We purchased our plane tickets. Grandma Nell arrived to care for Nick.

Micah, Del and I, arrived in Houston by plane on July 21st, 1993. We walked out of the airport terminal into what felt like a blast furnace. My lungs were challenged by the heat, unable to suck enough oxygen out of the thick, moist air. We loaded our luggage into a cab, trying to acclimate. Micah looked as unsure of our new surroundings as I felt.

113

A social worker at Oakland Children's Hospital had made reservations for us at a Ronald McDonald House near Ketchell Hospital. The facility offered rooms for cancer victims and their families for a minimal fee. Driving there in a taxi, I felt humbled and near tears. When Micah was little, I went with Nick and him to the grand opening of the McDonald's restaurant in Sonora. We met Ronald. It was a big deal for both the boys. Each time we visited McDonald's they collected my change and dropped it in the Ronald McDonald House donation box near the cash register, never imagining those funds might someday benefit us. Standing at the doorway of that same House, I could barely speak and was nervous about going inside.

Charity is a multifunctional word. It means many things: a *provision of help or relief to the poor. A fund established to help the needy. Benevolence or generosity toward others or toward humanity. Indulgence or forbearance in judging others.* Most of us imagine charity as something we do, a voluntary donation going 'out' to the community: *outstretched* arms, an *outpouring* of money, an *outreach, out* of compassion, *out* of love. Switching gears, readjusting your mindset to *accept* rather than to *give* can cause confusion, similar I would imagine to changing religions, moving to a different country where the customs, ideologies are different from your own. Walking through the doors of the Ronald McDonald House was yet another step into a world that previously had been untraveled, one where pride took a back seat. Though I was finally beginning to understand that we were not alone in our journey, my voice still reflected humility. "Hello," I said timidly. "We have a reservation?"

"Oh, hello! We've been expecting you. Welcome!

We're glad you're here." The woman who greeted us was kind and friendly. She explained the House rules, showed us the facility and our room. We had just enough time to wash our faces and freshen up before Micah's scheduled clinic visit. Back in a taxi, Micah and I held hands, looking out the window at the streets and buildings surrounding Ketchell Hospital, trying to get a feeling for where we were and where we were going.

Ketchell Hospital was located in the center of a medical complex occupying several city blocks. As we climbed out of the taxi and faced the hospital, I felt the same apprehension, the same dread as when we first visited Oakland Children's Hospital two years earlier. Foreign. It all felt so foreign. "It's okay," I said, reassuring myself as much as Micah. He stood close to me, looking at everything with anxious eyes, fearful of the unknown but eager to get the job done.

"Mom, look," he said, turning away. I saw what Micah saw, recoiling with him. Several patients stood in front of the hospital, but two caught our attention with undeniable morbidity. A woman with a bulbous red nose and with chunks of her lower lip missing was standing beside her IV pole, being fed chemotherapy through a Broviac similar to Micah's. It was not the way she looked that upset him; it was that she was smoking, inhaling deeply the cigarette smoke that most likely caused her cancer. The second patient -- a man -- was also smoking, but through a hole in his throat. The cigarette hung in the hole like a loaded gun, passing death into his lungs by a circumvented route. The sight of denial induced illness, a person mindfully choosing death over life, was more than Micah could tolerate. He got

115

tearful and angry. I could see in his face, his desire to yell at them, to say all the things I was thinking as well. *"What are you doing? Are you crazy? Stop that! Stop it now!"*

Micah looked at me and whispered, "I don't like it here. It's not like Oakland."

I put my arm around him and leaned down close to his ear. "It's okay," I told him. "Let's meet with Dr. Klu. You're not committed to anything, Micah. If you don't feel comfortable, if you want to go home, just tell me; we'll talk about this later and make a decision as a family, okay?" Micah nodded and gripped my hand tighter. We hurried through the sliding glass doors and on to the clinic, checked in with the receptionist and waited.

A nurse called Micah's name, and led us to an examining room. She took Micah's temperature, checked his blood pressure, pulse rate, height and weight. Dr. Klu came in with Micah's chart in hand, photocopied paperwork from Oakland Children's Hospital. He introduced himself to Del and me, and then to Micah. When he asked questions, he asked them of me; his eyes were directed at me when he spoke, so different from Debbie and Tom, from Dr. Feusner and Dr. Beach. Micah stiffened and looked offended. Dr. Klu was using expressions like, "When *he* goes for a dental exam; When *he* has his feet checked; When *he* has his eyes examined.

"Please speak to Micah," I told him. "He's used to his doctors addressing him directly."

"Oh, I'm sorry," Dr Klu said, patting Micah on the leg. He flipped to a new page in Micah's chart. "Yes, I see a note from Dr. Beach. It seems that Micah has been active in his treatment, is that right?" This time he looked at

116

Micah and smiled.

Micah nodded his head. "I like to know what's going on," he said. "And be involved in decisions regarding my body."

"Okay then. Micah, I've gone over your latest test results, and I agree with Dr. Beach. We need to get you ready for transplant as soon as possible. According to your latest lab work, eighty-five percent of your blood cells are abnormal. Your blast count is very high."

My lips tingled, and I shivered. Micah glanced at me, watching for my reaction. His elevated blast count was the first thing I had intentionally kept from him. Delays had cost him nearly six weeks; to most people, six weeks seem like a breezy succession of days within the span of a year, but for Micah those six weeks became an imposed life sentence, had given his leukemia a chance to gain more of a foothold, his blast count to rise beyond what was manageable. I fought to keep my thoughts focused, to remain clear-headed.

"We'll start today," Dr. Klu said. "Micah, we'll be checking everything from your teeth to your toenails."

"Micah's always had good teeth," I said, realizing right away how foolish that must have sounded.

"Mom, do you remember when Nick spit in Dr. Jon's face?" Micah said, chuckling.

I did remember, and Micah's chuckling was the only thing that seemed right at that moment. It felt good to laugh with him. Micah loved his dentist. Dr. Jon Parker had seen both my boys since they each were two years old. At Nick's first dental examination, Dr. Jon told him to spit, so he did, not understanding that Dr. Jon meant to spit into

117

the stainless steel bowl at the side of the dentist chair. Micah had comforted Nick ahead of time, telling him how great Jon Parker was, and that he should do just as Dr. Jon told him to do during the examination. So Nick did, spewing water into Dr. Jon's face, to the shock of everyone in the room; Micah, me, Dr. Jon's assistant, Dr. Jon. We all had a good laugh.

Dr. Klu examined Micah's mouth, his teeth. "Your mouth looks good," he said. "No mouth sores, no cavities that I can see. Still, we'll have our dental specialist take a look." He probed Micah's neck with his fingers, looked in his ears, checked his skin for rashes, bruises. "On the 23rd," he continued, "we'll begin preparation for the transplant itself. We'll start you on your chemo, begin your radiation treatments. When you're ready, Dad will undergo his part of this procedure. Del," he said, turning to Del, "while Micah's getting his pre-transplant checkups, we'll be doing the same to you, checking your health, doing preliminary lab work, okay?"

"Okay, Del said," rubbing his hands together. "I'm ready. Let's get this show on the road." He looked at Micah, and smiled.

We stayed at Ketchell Hospital until 5:00 p.m., doing just as Dr, Klu said, getting Micah's eyes checked, his ears, nose, throat, teeth, and feet. He had stomach and chest x-rays, a sonogram of his heart, lab work to check his liver enzymes, and kidney function. Del underwent the same types of examinations, and we met up at the end of the day, tired, hungry, ready to get out of the hospital for a while. For dinner, we decided on a restaurant recommended by the staff at the Ronald McDonald house. We made it a

118

celebration. Micah chose a sirloin steak and shrimp, a baked potato, and a big green salad, eating more than he had for a long while. He even asked for dessert, a hot fudge sundae with whipped cream and a cherry on top. After so many months of barely eating, Del and I smiled at each other, pleased with his effort and his appetite. He was nervous, but seemed happy, and hopeful. "We're doing the right thing," he assured us. "This is it. I can feel it."

We were to check in to the hospital at 7:00 a.m. the next morning, so back at the Ronald McDonald House, we passed on offers to enjoy communal television or play games with other families who were staying there. Quiet sounded best at that point. Being together, being alone, was what we needed most. After phoning Nick, and Grandma Nellie, we fell into a restless sleep.

That next morning, while Del waited with Micah in the hospital admissions office, I spoke with the admissions coordinator. "We've come up with an estimate of cost for Micah's transplant," she said, "but of course, it could be a great deal more than this." She pushed a sheet of paper across the desk. At the bottom of a typed column listing bare minimum procedures, the total read $168,000.00. "Is there any way," she asked, "that you can make another payment toward Micah's account at this time?"

"No! I can't make another payment! The money I sent you is all that we have! You agreed to do this for $108,000.00." I checked the tone of my voice and relaxed my shoulders, aware that Micah could see me, that his head was angled in my direction, watching my facial expressions, aware of my body language.

"Yes, we agreed to the $108,000.00 for a down

119

payment, but we need to know that you have a plan in place for the balance," the admissions coordinator said. "Have you talked any further with your insurance carrier?"

"Not since we left California. And I have no other plan in place, but I'll work on it from here, from the hospital. Please. I can't worry about this now. I need to get back to my son."

"I understand, yes. I'll send a representative up to Micah's room in a couple of days to see how things are progressing."

We were given directions to the Children's Transplant Unit, wound our way through a maze of hallways, up an elevator to the correct floor and to the nurse's station. We introduced ourselves and were led to Micah's hospital room, already aware of an environment far different from the one we were used to at Oakland Children's Hospital. There was no Debbie and there was no Tom. The nurses at Ketchell Hospital were all business. No tender touches. No jokes or attempts to get to know Micah on any level other than professional. There was a rush to get things done, an understandable urgency in the mannerisms of everyone around. "I wish Debbie was here," Micah whispered. "They don't do anything the way they did at Oakland."

The nervous concern in Micah's face reminded me of the day he started first grade. At some point during his kindergarten year, he had fallen in love with his teacher. Pam Oakes had made the transition from being at home to being at school an easy one. Micah loved everything about her. She was warm and cuddly, just like me. She was kind, thoughtful, and considerate of everyone's feelings, like Debbie at Oakland Children's. As I walked him into his first grade classroom on that first day of school in August of 1986, dressed in new clothes, with his new backpack and lunch pail, he lasted about ten seconds, came running out the door after me crying, "Don't leave me here, Momma! Please, I want Mrs. Oakes! Don't leave me here, *please!*" In the transplant unit at Ketchell Hospital, Micah had that same expression on his face, was pleading just as dramatically with his eyes. I could not help but smile at him and pray that it would be the same as it was back then, that he would eventually fall as much in love with these new nurses as he had with his first grade teacher, Mrs. Chapman.

As usual, Micah's feelings echoed my own. His Broviac care was handled differently: nurses placed the syringes, alcohol pads, gauze, and tape on the bedspread rather than on a surgical drape as we had been taught so meticulously to do at Oakland Children's Hospital. A nurse on the late night shift dropped a syringe on the floor, picked it up, removed the cap, intending to use it anyway to flush Micah's catheter. "Oh no," he said. "Nurse Tom wouldn't allow that. You need to get a new one. Throw that one away, please." As I agreed with him, reiterating his concern, we both got a dirty look as the nurse shook her head in disagreement. "The cap is still on the syringe," she said. "It's fine, really."

"I'm sure you're right," I said. "But please, this is all new to us, and we're used to being cautious. Can you just get a new syringe?"

"Different hospitals have different protocols," she said. "We may not do things exactly as you're used to, but we'll take good care of you. Relax."

Micah rolled his eyes. I looked at Del, and we both

chuckled nervously. I felt an uncharacteristic attitude slide into place, as I looked around the room. The pumps and IV poles looked the same as at Oakland. The same beep, beep chimed, announcing an empty bag of fluids. The room was clean and nice. There was a window seat, a scrub sink, a bathroom, a closet. I looked outside toward the nurse's station. Unlike Oakland, there were no children in the hallway. There were no volunteers holding babies. There were no clowns, no classrooms, or teen lounges. The descriptive phrase that came to me at that moment was 'urgent care professionalism'. All business. Big business. Urgent care.

On the 23rd of July, Dr. Klu began administering chemotherapy to Micah; tiny white pills, larger orange ones, and an IV drip set to run over a course of five days. Micah's counts dropped quickly; isolation rules were put into effect -- masks, gloves, no physical contact with bare hands. At night, I lay watching my son -- so quiet, so still. Nothing passed by me, not an involuntary jerk of an arm, nor an attempt to roll over through the mass of the tubal spaghetti that was attached to his chest. I saw every breath, heard every whimper, each interruption, every nurse entering the room to administer medication or draw Micah's blood or check his pumps; there were four of them now, beeping away simultaneously into the night.

Micah was assigned a social worker and a patient advocate. They each came to his hospital room, explaining their positions and offering assistance as their jobs allowed. I asked the patient advocate to intervene with the financial coordinators, to answer their questions, and assure them I was doing my best. I needed my focus to stay on Micah.

The mounting issue of no medical coverage was fighting for prioritized space in my already crowded brain. Placing part of this responsibility in the hands of a professional allowed a temporary solution. The social worker suggested I contact the Texas Department of Human Services to see if they might offer any assistance. She was kind enough to act as a go-between, providing her office phone and fax machine for my personal use. She even hand-delivered responses to Micah's room.

Texas Department of Human Services
RE: Micah Chase % Shelley Chase
NOTIFICATION OF INELIGIBILITY

1. You do not qualify for Medicaid at this time. If your circumstances change, you may reapply.
2. You are not eligible for TP11-Three Month Prior. Reason: "You do not meet residence requirements for assistance."

During a phone conversation pertaining to this denial, a nice woman from the Texas Department of Human Services informed me that if I were alone and an indigent, Micah would get his transplant free of charge. If I had arrived in Houston three months earlier, declared myself single and in need of welfare, I would have received all the help I needed. Under those circumstances my children would automatically qualify for health care in the state of Texas. If I were an immigrant in need of subsidized care, if Micah were abandoned, if, if, if...

Also at the social worker's suggestion, I phoned the California Children's Services in San Francisco and requested an application for emergency financial assistance.

The people involved with CCS had been especially helpful with information and offers of relevant services when we were at Oakland Children's Hospital. It was a long shot, I knew. CCS was, after all, a California based organization. By the next day, I had an official response:

NOTICE OF ACTION
CALIFORNIA CHILDREN SERVICES
CHILDREN'S MEDICAL SERVICES

Dear parents of Micah Chase:
Your application for CCS is denied. The reason for this action is: CCS can only accept a request for bone marrow transplant from an approved transplant center, according to our regulations.

CCS Program Director

Not an approved transplant center, by whose standards, I wondered? My thoughts flashed backwards to conversations between the doctors at Oakland Children's and the doctors at the transplant center at UCSF, conversations between the doctors at UCSF and doctors at transplant centers in Los Angeles, New York, and Ketchell Hospital in Houston, all top-notch facilities with experience and documented successes. Was this just a Catch 22, a matter of state-to-state noncompliance? If so, how could this be? I had paid taxes, both federal and state, since I was sixteen years old. For the first time in my life, I felt as if I lived in a land separated by borders, as if there were invisible boundaries across state lines. It went against everything I had been taught and believed in, yet there it was, stretched in front of me as daunting and pointedly secure as a barbed wire fence. I faxed a letter back to CCS, pleading with them to reconsider. Ketchell Hospital may not have been an approved transplant center, according to CCS criteria, but it was considered one of the top facilities in the country. I was no longer sure what the basis for approval of a transplant center would be, but surely the patient and his doctor's recommendations should be taken into account. The way I understood it, CCS was set up to help children in Micah's condition overcome their medical challenges, regardless of how 'risky' the procedure. To deny a child that chance was defeating the purpose for which the organization was initiated in the first place.

Rather than wait for a response, I phoned CCS. The woman I spoke with was apologetic but explained that her hands were tied. She spoke with great regret, explaining in detail the bylaws of CCS. In order to qualify for financial assistance, she told me, we would have to be in an 'approved transplant center,' in other words, a center located within the state of California. "I'm so sorry," she said. "If there was something I could do..."

Her empathy, her kindness, at least, meant something. I knew, without question, this woman would have pulled any strings she could, if there were any chance of changing the outcome of the CCS determination for denial.

Those first couple of nights Del and I stayed in Micah's hospital room, but we needed to be realistic; Micah would soon be in isolation and the rules were going to get much stricter. Only one parent would be allowed to spend the night, and even that was with special permission. We were a long way from home and needed a place where we could nap, shower and change clothes. The Ronald McDonald

House had provided an immediate solution, but we needed to find something more secure and long-term. Micah's patient advocate told us about a woman who often shared her home with the families of patients at Ketchell Hospital. Del met with our perspective host and was impressed by her compassion, her understanding of our situation. He said her home was close by and in an old-fashioned neighborhood where we could walk, think and spend time recuperating from the rigors of Micah's hospitalization, if need be. The house had a guestroom with its own entryway and attached bathroom. He thought it would be a great situation for us and convinced me that taking the room would be a good move.

Del would stay at Pat's at night, and I would sleep in a sleeper chair in Micah's room. During the day, at some point, I would go for a shower and fresh change of clothes while Del stayed with Micah. We had seen too many things, watched too many mistakes made throughout Micah's care to do otherwise. On that point, we were insistent. Even at Oakland Children's, where patient care was of utmost priority, mistakes were made. Doctors and nurses were human. The staff in the cafeteria, the maintenance crew, all were human, and mistakes were made -- moldy bread on a sandwich for lunch, syringes left on a freshly mopped floor, an accidentally skipped dose of chemotherapy. One of us would be in the room with Micah at all times. It was a pact Del and I made early on.

The radiation part of the treatment was tough. Micah was deeply saddened by the explanations of the after effects he would suffer. "Unfortunately," the radiologist told him, "total body radiation has a profound effect. You won't be

126

able to have children, Micah, not the usual way." The look in Micah's eyes was desperate; his body shook, his head dropped to my chest. We sobbed softly together for a while, each of us recognizing the permanency behind the statement.

I held Micah's hand as he lay on a table in the radiation room, watching a radiologist draw lines and X's on his body with a black permanent pen. When the radiologist had finished, I kissed Micah and assured him I would wait just outside. Behind thick, protective walls, I could hear the giant machine grind and rumble as Micah got his treatment. I could feel the room vibrate under its awesome power. Minutes felt like hours. Whatever they were doing in there was affecting the guts of the building, the guts of my son. I stood up and paced the floor, feeling as if I might lose my balance due to the sway of my emotions. Burning, there was burning, I could sense it, smell it. Suddenly I understood the X's and the lines, the rumbling grind, the vibration beneath my feet: *You won't be able to have children, Micah, not the usual way.*

I struggled to compose myself as Micah came out of the x-ray room in a wheelchair, pushed by a smiling technician. "He did great," the technician said. "He's a real trooper." Micah smiled a half-grin, reached out for a hug, talking in a singed and shaky voice, "That wasn't so bad, Mom," he said. "I'm okay, really, I am," he reassured me.

My son, my protector, always. *'You are my sunshine, my only sunshine, please don't take my sunshine away'* I sang to myself. *Dear God, protect my child,* I prayed.

As Micah slept after his radiation treatment, I wrote another letter to our insurance company, listing the same

127

details as before, but this time, my wording was more urgent. It was faxed as a high priority to Dr. Bustoff and to the head of his corporate office:

"Because of your hesitancy and regardless of letters and phone calls stating the urgency of the situation, we have lost valuable time. Micah's condition has deteriorated, and he could wait no longer. We are in Houston now, and he is having his transplant. As far as your denial of his medical treatment, we will follow whatever measures we need to follow, including but not limited to finding an attorney who will help us settle this matter. If Micah had remained at Oakland Children's Hospital and continued on chemotherapy, his bills would have equaled or exceeded the cost quoted for this transplant. Please reconsider this matter, and think of this 'case' as a vital, loving child rather than a $ sign."

As the radiation and chemotherapy treatments continued, Micah grew homesick. We phoned Nick and Grandma Nellie every evening to check in and tell them we loved them. Micah wasn't feeling well enough to talk to friends, but he always perked up for Nick. "I miss my brother," he told me. "Can't Nick come here for a visit?" Del and I talked it over and decided it would be good for both Micah and Nick if we could figure out the logistics of such a trip. I spoke with my sister Jan. "We'll just do it," she said. She suggested she drive our car out, knowing it would make things easier if we had our own transportation while in Houston. "I can drive my car, and John can drive yours. There will be plenty of room for everyone, Nick and Grandma, Season and Levi, and if we come now, we'll be able to see Micah while he's still well enough to have visitors."

"Make the trip fun," I told her. "This has all been so

128

hard on Nick. Stop at the Grand Canyon. Mom's never been, and I've always wanted to take the kids."

"Shelley, you should save that trip," she said. "Take Micah and Nick yourself when Micah's better."

"No, I said. "I want you to go."

The Grand Canyon was a special place to me. I had taken two treks down into and through the Canyon, once on foot, once by raft. The rafting experience was one I swore I would do again and share with my boys someday. As I thought about Nick seeing it for the first time without me, I felt sad but thankful that he would be with my sister and his cousins. I was glad that he would experience something so peaceful and surreal, so timeless and spiritual before coming to Houston and seeing Micah. The Grand Canyon was a place that might give him strength and hope, some definition of the way life changes and flows with the passing of time. "I want you to go," I told Jan again. "Please. It would be good for all of you."

They arrived in Houston on July 28th. The familiarity of family in a place so far from home was a boost for all of us. Micah's counts had dropped substantially, however, and the doctors felt it best if his visitors were limited, so Nick, Grandma Nellie, and Auntie Jan were the only ones allowed up to his room. Season cried, trying to understand how it could possibly be best for Micah if she stayed away. Levi listened intently to our explanation of Micah's situation, nodding his head, trying to be brave. The following day, Jan, John, Season, and Levi left for home. Nick and Grandma Nellie stayed in Houston. They would live at Pat's house for the next two weeks and then fly home to California with Del if all went well during transplant and

129

after.

On July 29th, Del underwent his part of the procedure. In a few hours, he was back in Micah's room sleeping off the anesthesia on the day bed by the window. Dr. Klu came and spoke with me. "Everything went beautifully," he said. "You're husband will be sore for a few days, but there should be no side-effects other than that. His marrow should be ready for transplant just a little after midnight."

Under normal conditions, there would have been a final battery of tests. If the money had been available weeks earlier there would have been time to check for compatibility, but there wasn't. There would be no Petri-dish in which to view the possibilities, no team meetings to discuss the options because there were no options to discuss. Micah put a big red circle around the day: July 30th, 1993. "MY BONE MARROW TRANSPLANT," he wrote beside the date.

MICAH CHARLES CHASE
AN AUTOBIOGRAPHY
by Micah Chase (1992)

"I was born on a snowy morning, January 18, 1979 at 6:26 a.m. at the Sonora Community Hospital in Sonora, California.

My first words were Mama, Dada, kitty, and doggie. I took my first step on December 17, 1979. After that, my mom said I was able to climb over anything. I even climbed over a big barrier she made and took a walk by myself down our driveway before I was two.

When I was two, I went to the ocean for the first time. It must have been quite a trip, because I have loved the ocean ever since. On October 20, 1981, I had a new baby brother. We named him Nicholas. That was a great day in my life. As long as I can remember, I wanted a baby brother.

In September of 1985, I entered kindergarten at Belleview School. I was very excited. I was also frightened because I had never been in school before. In the first grade, I went on a family vacation for about a week. We reached Kingman Arizona, where my Grandpa had a heart attack and died. This affected me greatly, as I loved my grandpa very much. He was very special to me. We had a great relationship. I didn't go to school for about a week after that.

In 1987 I went into the second grade and I got involved in Campfire Kids. My mom was our leader and we had meetings at my house. It was great. That year I also joined my first baseball team. Actually, it was a tee-ball team and our name was the Bobcats. In 1988, I entered the third grade. I played tee-ball again that year. In the third grade, I was in a play called 'Let George Do it'. We went to different schools to perform it. Also in 1988, we had a Japanese Exchange student stay at our house for six weeks. Her name was Kimiyo. She showed me a lot of things including origami. I entered a talent show in 1988, too, with my friends Mike Jacobson and Austin

131

Cripps. We had a great time. That summer, my family took a trip to Death Valley. It was very hot but very beautiful. If you can believe it, we found a swimming pool in the middle of the desert! I think that pool saved our lives!

In the fourth grade, I went on an overnight fieldtrip to Monterey with my class. My mom came as a chaperone. It was really fun. We went to the aquarium and to the tide pools. It was cool because I had been there before and could show my friends some really neat stuff, like sea urchins and sea cucumbers. That same year, I took a trip to Yellowstone National Park with my family. I went to Montana, Wyoming, and Idaho. It was awesome. I saw elk, moose, and buffalo. We saw Old Faithful and went to some great but smelly hot springs.

In the summer before sixth grade, my baseball team went to Stockton because we won all of our games in Tuolumne County. We played in the Tournament of Champions. In 1990, I entered the sixth grade, and won second place in an essay contest for all of Tuolumne County. It was on the drought.

After sixth grade, in the summer before seventh grade, I was rushed to Oakland Children's Hospital because of low blood counts. It was four weeks in the hospital before I was diagnosed with Myleodysplastic Syndrome, a rare form of leukemia. I missed out on the whole summer, and the first quarter of seventh grade. I was able to go to school for the last three quarters of the year though, and I've been doing most everything I want, and having a pretty normal life, so far. My parents are really good about that. They keep me safe, but let me have a happy life. My brother is always supportive of me. My friends are awesome. My best friend Jason is always there when I need to talk or just have fun. I feel very lucky.

Chapter 11

The transplant was administered just like a blood transfusion. Del's healthy pink marrow hung in a bag from an IV pole and was pumped through a clear plastic tube into Micah's Broviac, his veins, and into the heart of his bones. Things went more smoothly and quickly than expected, and the transplant team seemed happy. As planned, I stayed with Micah while Del recuperated, sleeping nights at Pat's house. Over the next few days, Micah slept a lot. He ate nothing and drank very little. He was weak and shaky, but insisted on bathing himself, getting himself to the restroom, and spending a little time in the chair by the window seat. He did his routine mouth care -- applying special toothpaste to his teeth and gums with a soft sponge, rinsing, swishing, rinsing again. I read to him chapters of a book we had brought from home: *Whalesong* by Robert Siegel. We played cards and watched television. I talked, and he pretended to listen, appeasing me with a smile or by nodding his head. We played the Imagine Game. *"Mama, just imagine...we're at the ocean...we're in Hawaii...we're home."*

At night, I kept the promise I had made to him, waking each time a nurse came in to check his vital signs, asking questions, acting as his advocate, being his mother, always.

133

In those long hours, there was a lot of time to reflect. It was not hard to picture Micah as he looked when he was a baby. While sleeping, he still had that angelic face, those perfectly formed brows, long lashes. His lips still puckered in that cute little way, sending fish kisses around the room and into my heart. I could feel a tingling in my breasts and imagined them full of milk. I closed my eyes and saw myself nursing him, remembering how I would rock him for hours afterward, letting him nap in my arms rather than in his crib, mesmerized by the feel of his little body curled against mine, being in love with the naturally sweet smell of his skin.

Memories, like reels of silent picture footage, ran through my mind: of Micah and Nick sitting on the hearth beside the fireplace at home, eating chicken soup and homemade tortillas, building a fort out of blankets spread across the living room furniture, stocking it with flashlights, comic books, and their brand new Care Bears. I relived moments of tenderness from my childhood: my mother rubbing my neck and chest with warm Vicks VapoRub when I was sick, making me a cup of hot chocolate or tea as I sat snuggled in blankets in a gold fabric reclining chair. I remembered other mothers I had met over the years: a woman who came to my elementary school every day during my fourth grade year to bring her daughter medication for her asthma, the mother of a friend of mine in high school who'd had an emotional breakdown after losing her youngest son in an automobile accident. I thought of a man I had met at Oakland Children's Hospital, a father who had shaved his head bald, swearing he would go without hair until his son finished his chemotherapy and had hair again. I remembered the same man coming into Micah's room one night with a petition, asking for my signature, my support in his effort to improve the food served to the children in the hospital. "It's what we do," he told me. "As the parents of sick kids, it's our responsibility to protect their rights. As a parent, we do for them what we can. It's all we can do. It's the only thing there is." I recalled the sadness in his eyes that night, the depth of his fatherly concern. As time passed and his son got sicker, his eyes grew more desperate, his demands became more intense. Some weeks he would come in Micah's room every night, to talk, to vent, and to cry. If his reasons were not entirely clear to me at Oakland Children's Hospital, at Ketchell Hospital in Houston, they made perfect sense. As a parent, when you are scared, when you feel powerless, helpless, you do the only things you can do: you gather signatures on a petition to register complaints about hospital food; you make sure all Broviac dressing supplies are kept sterile and that dressing changes are done properly; you watch to see that the nurse who is caring for your child is gentle, sensitive to his needs, to his dignity.

In the daytime, Del and I fell into a routine of watching and waiting. We would talk about lab results; note Micah's skin color, the way he moved, spoke, his emotional sensitivity. We took turns going down to the cafeteria for food, neither of us able to stay away for long, both of us feeling anxious, guilty almost, for eating when Micah could not keep anything down. We strained our ears, trying to listen to the conversations of Micah's transplant team out in the hallway, their discussions of his progress, his medications, his body's response to the transplant.

135

Our new friend Pat, the woman who opened her heart and her Houston home to my family, was drawn to Nick, welcoming him as if he were her own, listening to his needs, his fears regarding his brother, telling him how strong and brave he was. She kept him busy playing on her trampoline and in her yard as Grandma Nellie learned to navigate the city streets to and from the hospital. When Micah was in isolation, neither Grandma Nellie nor Nick could visit, so they took little side trips, visiting shopping malls and parks, keeping busy, staying active.

Two weeks after the transplant Micah's counts rose appropriately, and isolation rules were lifted. Nick and Grandma came to visit, telling Micah stories about the things he would get to see and do once he was out of the hospital. Del and I removed our protective masks and took short walks with Micah down the hall past the nurse's station. Since things were going so well, Del made plans to go home. He booked three flights from Houston to San Francisco for the end of the week. Nick, Grandma Nellie, and I drove to Galveston on the day before they were due to leave, went to the beach, walked and talked. Leaving Micah that morning was difficult, but my time with Nick was crucial. Del was with Micah, and their time alone together was just as important since we weren't sure how long it would be before Del could come back to Houston.

I drove them to the airport and said goodbye at the terminal. Nick promised to call me as soon as he got home. As we hugged and kissed, I thought of all the times I'd had to leave him over the past two years, all the shuffling around, the uncertainty of our lives. Just as with Micah, Nick's grief had taken a toll. I could see it in his eyes. I

136

could feel it in the strength of his goodbye hug.

In the melancholy that followed their leaving, Micah and I tried to lift each other's spirits by discussing the next steps in his recuperation. Pat had assured me that we could stay with her after Micah was released from the hospital, and she asked about the possibility of having Nick move to Houston, letting him start sixth grade there when the time was right. Since Del and I had discussed this possibility beforehand, it was a relief to know that such a crucial piece of our plan was potentially in place.

The following day, the hospital's financial coordinator came to check on my progress toward the payment of Micah's bills. I had no progress to report but assured her that I was following every lead that came my way. Two days later she came again. I noticed Micah flinch and saw his body slump when she spoke in front of him about the need for "expediency in the matter". I went to see his patient advocate, voicing my concern. Micah had other things on his mind, like getting well and staying strong. Simply hearing that there was a major push by the hospital to assure payment of his bills had stressed him.

Four weeks after transplant, Micah developed a rash. The doctors increased the level of steroids he was receiving in hopes of warding off the graft versus host disease they perceived to be the cause of the problem. As the medication was increased, he developed other symptoms such as mental confusion and jaundice. It was hard to tell whether the symptoms were getting worse because of the graft versus host or because of the increased dosages of his medications. From one day to the next, he would go from better to worse to better again, his body bouncing like a tired little salmon, fighting to make its way upstream.

I tried to stay calm and focused, but I'd had so little sleep it was hard to keep those parts of myself awake and alert. As Micah's condition worsened, I thought again about the father I had met at Oakland Children's Hospital, the anguish I saw in his eyes when his son's life was in danger of being lost. I remembered his words: *"As the parents of sick kids, it's our responsibility to protect their rights. As a parent, we do for them what we can. It's all we can do. It's the only thing there is."*

My ears became keen to conversations in the hallway, my frazzled senses sending me into a flurry of anger one afternoon as Dr. Klu spoke to his interns. "He's had fifteen bowel movements today," he told them, chuckling as he examined Micah's chart. I leaned over Micah, making sure he was asleep, and then walked into the hallway, confronting Dr. Klu. "If he was awake, he could have heard you," I said, my voice shaking. "Please," I begged, "don't discuss these things where he can hear you!" I turned away as he apologized, feeling violated and alone. *As a parent, we do for them what we can. It's all we can do. It's the only thing there is.* Tears rolled down my cheeks. I wanted to speak with Del, to tell him what had happened. I wanted to talk to Dr. Beach, to tell her the humiliation that had been put upon the little boy she had cared for so greatly. I wanted to scream and yell, to curse Dr. Klu, to blame him. Instead, I went to Micah, sat beside him on his bed, and rubbed his legs; I sang one of his favorite Bon Jovi *songs:*

"Hello, again, it's you and me, kinda always like it used to be, sippin' wine, killing time, trying to solve life's mysteries. How's your

life, it's been a while, God it's good to see you smile. I see you reaching for your keys, looking for a reason not to leave.

"If you don't know if you should stay, if you don't say what's on your mind, baby, just breathe, there's nowhere else tonight we should be. You wanna make a memory?

"I dug up this old photograph. Look at all that hair we had. It's bittersweet to hear you laugh. Your phone is ringing, I don't wanna ask. If you go now, I'll understand. If you stay, hey, I've got a plan. We're gonna make a memory. You wanna steal a piece of time, you can sing the melody to me, and I can write a couple of lines? You wanna make a memory?

"If you don't know if you should stay, and you don't say what's on your mind...

"Baby, just breathe."

Hearing his favorite song sung in my raspy voice woke Micah up, made him smile and snuggle closer. As off-key as it might have sounded to anyone else, hearing the familiar tune gave him comfort, and that was enough reason to sing it again and again, softly, and then in a whisper, to take him back to the edge of sleep.

Chapter 12

As the days crept by, Micah grew more agitated. He couldn't put words together into sentences that made sense, but the confusion in his eyes told me more than I wanted to know. I stayed by his bedside, rarely leaving his room. I sang old tunes we had sung together when he was small, told the stories he loved to hear when he was little, talked about his cousins, his friends, and Nick. I spoke about anything that would keep him connected to me and to the purpose of our trip to Houston, to getting well, and going home when this was over. I reminded him of the kind of kid he was, the kind of man he had become in such a short time. I told him how proud I was to be his mother. I begged him to stay strong.

Time lost its balance. My mind distorted with the reality of Micah's condition. Amid a flurry of activity, a young boy, another transplant patient who was suffering the same side effects as Micah, was sent to a different hospital for dialysis and supplementary treatments. In a conversation with his mother, I learned that his family was from Texas and that they were well insured. Her son had the same type of transplant as Micah, and there was never a question regarding coverage or payment of medical bills. I started imagining the worst. If we had insurance, I wondered, would the situation be different? Would Micah be sent out for dialysis, would he be given more options, would the doctors be taking things further if money had been available up front? *As a parent, we do for them what we can. It's all we can do. It's the only thing there is.*

All of a sudden, it was August 30th, and my son was slipping away. My children were my life; half of all that I had ever wanted was lying in a hospital bed, still as stone. Dr. Klu told me that I had better call Del back to the hospital. "What are you saying? Are you telling me, Micah isn't going to make it?" I sobbed.

"I'm sorry," Dr. Klu said. "It's not looking good." He looked straight at me. I could see the pain in his eyes. "We need to know your feelings," he asked, "about life support."

Del was back in Houston by nightfall. Decisions. We were asked to make decisions at a time when we could no longer make them. Tired and emotionally drained, we asked Dr. Klu one question. "Are you telling us you're ready to put him on life support?"

"Yes, I'm afraid that's what I'm saying. I'm sorry."

Del's face was haggard, distraught beyond the point of pain. We looked into each other's eyes, making sure, confirming the unthinkable. I took a deep breath, hesitating no longer than a moment to search the doctor's face once more, before words came out of my mouth I never imagined I would say. "Then no. No more tubes, no more pumps. No catheters or shots. Can you make him comfortable?"

"Yes."

From either side of Micah's bed, Del and I watched as

141

the web of plastic tubing was disconnected from our son. We watched as Micah slept.

I turned to Micah. I whispered his name and gently touched his face. He felt so cold. I asked him, begged him to squeeze my hand. I asked him if we had made the wrong decision.

His words came in a whisper, barely audible, but clear and in complete sentences for the first time in several days. "I love you, Mommy. I love you, Mommy," he said.

A ramshackle memory of one particular day, a month earlier in Sonora, came to mind: Micah had not been feeling well and was depressed about the delay of his transplant. We were outside when he fell to the ground and just lay there. I ran and tried to help him up, but he didn't move, wouldn't open his eyes. I realized then that he was acting out death, trying to imagine what it would be like, what it would feel like, to die. I got angry, and yelled at him. "Get up!" I screamed, unable to digest the importance of his act.

Micah never did like to go into anything unprepared.

I leaned over the rail that now guarded my son, pressing my forehead against Micah's cheek, preparing to have a last, private conversation. "Oh, Baby...I'm sorry. I love you so much."

"Mommy?" I had to strain now, to hear anything at all. "Mommy? Mommy? I love you." The last of his speech faded away, along with the glitter in his eyes, into all that was left for him that made sense -- mumblings from old to ancient -- animal-like noises of the night.

"Baby, just breathe," I whispered frantically. *Baby, just breathe.*

Micah's attempt at talking ended with a gentle, sweet,

final breath, and I let him go to his angels, to those who waited to guide him on the next leg of his journey. I looked at Del, searching his face for answers. Drifting, each in our own grief, we hoped for a miracle, waiting for God to change his mind, for Micah to open his eyes, believing for a moment that together we could make it happen, as parents we could make it happen, that love would make it happen. Del touched Micah's cheek. So pale. So gray. I took Micah's small hand and placed it in Del's larger one, then threw my head back and let out one long, low scream.

Chapter 13

I won't let them hurt you, I promise, Micah. Mommy's here!
Breathe for Mommy! Now Micah! Breathe! Occasionally, the
doctors, the nurses, their attempts at conversation, their
need for permissions and details reached through the fog,
pulling me out of my effort to stay with Micah, to sustain
the essence of him that hovered in the hospital room.

"No, I'm sorry, but we don't want an autopsy. Micah's
had enough cutting and poking and prodding. No." I said
again. "Please, no autopsy." The words sounded desperate
and lost in delirium. Everything around me was spiraling
out of control. Autopsies were a procedure requested by
the police, a family member when the cause of death was
undetermined. It was the examination and dissection of a
dead body, by a coroner, to discover the cause of death.
Did we have an autopsy performed on my father when he
died? I couldn't remember. *I couldn't remember.*

The rise and fall of my chest kept time with the sounds
around me, the swishing of the nurse's shoes as she walked
across the room, the tapping of Dr. Klu's pencil against his
clipboard. "So many kids could benefit from Micah's
experience," he said again. "If we could just go in and look
around, run some tests, we might be able to further our
efforts for pediatric bone marrow transplantation."

I listened, I did. But there is no logic to a grieving mother's thoughts. In my clear, rational mind, I knew what an autopsy could mean for countless other children, but my rational mind was not in control. *If I let them cut Micah, so fresh into death, will he feel it? Will he hurt?* I wondered. *If I let them take his vital organs, how will he come back to me?*

"No," Del said firmly, dismissing Dr. Klu's request with a wave of his hand. "No autopsy," he added, turning away.

It was a selfish choice, I knew, but an autopsy was *one more thing*, another invasion of Micah's body that neither Del nor I could handle. Micah was done. He'd had enough. I had seen it in his eyes before he closed them for the last time. From the first day of his diagnosis, he had been involved in all major decisions regarding his care and treatment. In my eyes, at that moment, saying no was the only act of respect we could grant our son. At that moment, in my heart, there was no other choice to make.

As Dr. Klu left the room, the nurse asked if we were ready to step outside as well, so she could clean Micah's body before we said our final goodbyes. I questioned her, saying I would like to stay, that it would mean a great deal if I could help. "It would be easier, really, if you waited outside," she told me.

With great regret, I followed Del out of the room, feeling that I was losing a blessed privilege, missing a ceremony I should have been responsible for from start to finish. My body screamed for quiet time, family time, *our time. This wasn't real, it wasn't happening!* None of it made any sense. Dying was something that happened to a pet, my dog Apple, Nick's hamster, our baby goat, after a problem with her birthing.

145

As a child, on my grandfather's ranch, he and I found a baby bird that had fallen from its nest. Despite our efforts to feed and care for the little robin, it died. We had a funeral. Grandpa told me that life could be hard, that dying happened. "The days in a man's life amount to no more than the flutter of a butterfly's wing or the shadow of a cloud as it passes over the land. They come and go that quickly. The important thing is not the length of time he spends; it's the path he walks while he's here," he said with a reassuring smile.

I stood in the hallway, unsure of what to do. It was hard to walk on legs that shook like Jello. The drapes in Micah's room were closed. The door was shut. I opened my mouth to speak to Del but only whimpered. We hugged, chests heaving, hearts ravaged, empty.

When the door finally swung open, we could see our son. "I'll leave you alone for a bit," the nurse said, exiting with a small garbage bag filled with Micah's gauze and tubes and left over medication.

Finally. Finally.

The room was clean, no clutter, no mess. Micah was beautiful, as always, so perfect, so still. The nurse had dressed him in a set of shorts and a t-shirt we'd brought from home. He lay on top of the bedspread, as if he were asleep. I sat beside him and rubbed his legs, refusing to let go. I searched the room with my eyes, feeling his spirit. *Where are you?* I asked.

Up in that corner?
Standing beside me?
Are you hugging me, Micah? I feel you!
Oh God, I feel you.

"Hello, again, it's you and me, kinda always like it used to be....How's your life, it's been a while, God it's good to see you smile."

"If you don't know if you should stay, if you don't say what's on your mind, baby, just breathe..."

Micah, I love you! I screamed inside. *Come back! Don't go! I'm sorry I couldn't fix it. I'm sorry I couldn't make it better!*

The phone rang. It was Jan Lekas. "He's gone," I mumbled, when I heard her voice.

"Go be with him," she cried. "I love you, Shell. We'll talk a little later, okay?" she promised.

Del was at Micah's feet, quiet, contemplative. "I need to call Nick," I said, hoarsely.

My fingers were numb, felt awkward as I dialed. I got the number wrong and dialed again.

When Nick picked up the phone, it was as if he already knew. His breathing was rough, jagged, as he said, "Hello?"

I stroked Micah's forehead as I talked with Nick. "He fought so hard," I said. "You'd have been proud. Micah loved you so much, Nick," I told him, between my sobs and his.

"I know," Nick said. "Mom? He asked. "How's Micah getting home? I mean, how..."

"We'll work that out. Don't worry, okay?"

"When?"

"I'll be there as soon as I can. By tomorrow night, I'll be home, okay? Honey, go give Grandma Nellie some great big hugs. You two take care of each other until I get there, okay?"

"She's crying too," Nick whispered.

"I know, Baby. I know."

"I'll take her outside to look at the stars."

"Thank you, Baby. I love you."

The nurses had allowed us our privacy, but they were getting anxious. Someone peeked in the door. The head nurse came in the room with a clipboard, taking notes, questioning us about arrangements. Was Micah to be cremated, she wondered, or was his body to be flown home, to California? Del and I couldn't think clearly. We couldn't speak more than a few jumbled words to each other, how could we make such a decision? This was our son! *How can I leave him? Will he find his way home?*

"They're waiting to transport him," the head nurse told us, checking her watch. "So when you feel ready..." She walked out of the room, but came back in, fingering the stethoscope around her neck. "Micah's social worker will be here shortly to discuss arrangements."

To discuss arrangements? Who's they? Who was waiting to transport my son?

Micah was born in the middle of a snowstorm, the worst Sonora had seen in years. "He's a keeper," the doctor told us. "Yes, he is," I agreed. We brought him home from the hospital bundled in a wool blanket, snug and warm, safe and secure. I called him Punky Doodle. Del called him Motorboat. We lived on a mountaintop. We had raised him right. "Please get him ready, we want to take him home, to Nick and to Butchy," I said, looking at Del for his approval. Del nodded his head, but didn't speak, couldn't deal with what came next. For the first time in Micah's life, we wouldn't be there to take care of him. We wouldn't be

148

there when he was lifted onto a gurney and transported downstairs. We wouldn't be there to make sure he was treated respectfully while being readied for his final journey home. My body quivered, but I fought back any tears. I looked around the room once more, hoping for a glimpse, some sign that he was there. Micah had to see that I could be strong. He had to know that I could turn and walk away. I leaned down and kissed him, and Del did the same.

In the hallway outside Micah's room, I hugged Dr. Klu, and thanked him for trying to save Micah's life. We spoke with the social worker about the arrangements to have Micah's body transported to a funeral parlor in Houston and then brought home. The hospital's financial coordinator also paid us a visit, clipboard in hand, with an *estimation* of what we owed the hospital, her latest *estimate* to date. She's quick, I thought. The *final* bill, the *finality* of a life. Would she have been so prompt had we been residents of Texas, if we were rich, if we were poor, if our insurance company had fulfilled their responsibility? The numbers blurred on the paper she held in front of my face. I signed blindly, as did Del, promising I would get in touch with her as soon as I could.

As a parent, we do for them what we can. It's all we can do. It's the only thing there is.

We left Micah's hospital room, walked down the hall past the nurse's station, got in the elevator, descended three stories and walked out of Ketchell Hospital into the muggy Houston air.

Blasted by the intense heat, I felt scattered, as if my feet were gone, my legs, separated from the rest of my body, as I struggled to find a new balance. A piece of me was in

149

California with Grandma Nellie; a piece of me was lying behind me in the hospital. Alone. We were all alone. I felt cheated, robbed of Micah's life, of the time he would have known me, as I had known my father, my grandfather; robbed of a future, of every song and story and life lesson we might have shared, every adventure we might have had, his loves, his joys, his heartaches.

In the years before my father died, he had a habit of throwing coins in the dirt, leaving Micah and Nick, Kip and Katy, Levi and Season thinking they were discovering lost treasure as they walked with him and Grandma Nellie along the canal bank near their home. Around the Thanksgiving table last year, the kids recalled those times with their grandfather, the love they had for him. Katy and Season never realized their Grandpa's deception, and I recalled the shocked look on their faces, the laughter that followed, when we told them about his habit of carrying quarters, dimes, and nickels in his pocket for the sheer joy of watching his grandchildren run to scoop them up. To the kids, the canal bank was a source of unending wealth, not only the money they found, but the time they spent with their grandparents.

My father's death was horrible, but Micah's death was worse. I was forty-three years old. The death of my child was a black hole that existed outside the limit of my life experience.

Back at Pat's house, I called my friend Terry. She screamed when I told her the news. I babbled while she cried. In my hands, I held a get-well card her daughter Jenny had sent Micah a week earlier:

Micah:

"Hey Stud, how are you doing? I hope you're doing okay. I think about you all the time. I'm gonna come and visit you. I miss ya and love ya

.

Love always, Jenny B/F/F!!!!"

Micah and Jenny had been friends since Kindergarten. When Micah was at Oakland Children's, Terry and Jenny came to visit. Once, on their way to the hospital, Terry saw a huge white limousine stopped at a convenience store. Out of the store came Muhammad Ali. Knowing that he was a favorite of Micah's, Terry spun a U-turn and was in hot pursuit as the limo drove away. They followed Mr. Ali to a restaurant, got his autograph, and a get well note, handwritten on a paper cocktail napkin. I remembered how the napkin, the story of Terry and Jenny chasing Muhammad Ali's limo, made Micah laugh. "Terry, only you would do something that crazy," he told her. "Thank you," he said. "This is so cool!"

Micah had so many friends, good friends, kids he had known all his life. Jason had been a constant support, as had his mother, Diane. Being a nurse, she had come over often to monitor potential problems: a rash around Micah's Broviac site, a suspicious sore on his leg, unexplained aching behind his eyes. Jason and Jenny, Mindy, Christina, Sarah, Brian, Jonathon, Chris and Caitie, Erik, Aaron, Shaylyn, Austin, and many others. I knew how Micah's death would affect them. I knew that Nick, Del, and I were not the only ones who would feel the pain of losing him. And his cousins, especially the ones who were so close -- Kip and Katy, Levi and Season, how will they ever get through this, I wondered.

My mind was on getting home, being with Nick, getting Micah to Sonora without incident. There was no point in trying to sleep. I called my sisters, the grandparents on Del's side of the family, aunts, uncles, and cousins. I phoned a teacher from Belleview School, my friend, Pam Oakes, and told her what had happened, asked her to inform the staff, the kids, somehow. Micah's friends were in high school now and would have support from the high school counselor, but Nick's friends, many of Micah's younger classmates, would need help dealing with our tragedy as well. Del and I got through the night by talking mindlessly, packing our things, saying goodbye to our host, Pat. Each word was laborious, the birthing of a life without Micah. Showering was tedious, a time to shed tears. How do you dress, comb your hair, look yourself in the mirror when the person you recognized as yourself is gone? How do you go on, when a huge piece of you has died?

Micah's social worker arranged the air flight for Micah and me on American Airlines, a nonstop trip from Houston to San Francisco. She contacted the funeral parlor in Sonora, requesting that they meet us at the plane and transport Micah from San Francisco to Sonora. My sisters, Jan and Carol, would pick me up at the airport.

Friends offered to fly out and drive our Toyota home from Texas, but Del was adamant that he do it, to have the time alone, to think, he said. He drove me to the airport in Houston, saw me to the American Airlines terminal and helped check my baggage. We stood apart as we said goodbye. His eyes were distant, already set on the road, it seemed. I sat down in the waiting area and watched him walk away, wondering if he would be okay -- if he would get lost in the canyons of Arizona or along the highways of Nevada -- if he would run away with his grief and never come home. There were people sitting in the seats next to me, walking past me, standing nearby, yet I was alone.

Once aboard, I sat in my seat with my son's body below me in the belly of the plane. I spoke to no one, was numb, thinking only of him, wondering if it was cold down there, if he was covered snuggly enough, if his spirit was with me in the cabin or flying free beside the plane like the Bald Eagles he loved. One thing Micah had wanted to do in the last months of his life was to fly, to hang glide tandem with a friend of mine who offered to take him if his doctors gave the okay. We were within weeks of making that happen when Micah's counts dropped dramatically, and the plans to go to Texas were initiated.

In the carry-on suitcase on my lap were Micah's extra clothes, books, pictures, a Nintendo Game Boy that had been given to him by his friend Brian. I pulled the game player out, manipulating the control buttons, placing my fingers where Micah's fingers had been just days before. Even in isolation, he had played to win, fighting dragons and shooting hoops from the confines of his bed. Around my neck was the medicine bag made for Micah by a Grandfather from the Tuolumne Band of Me-Wuk. I gripped the soft leather pouch, holding it next to my heart, feeling as if I was existing on some other plane of consciousness, watching the world go on around me through someone else's eyes.

Fall was normally filled with school and friends, quiet

153

walks along the old miner's ditch below our house, cherished talks with Micah and Nick. Someone once told me that Micah was an old spirit. He was precocious and fun loving but was wise beyond his years. He listened as well as he talked, hearing my words, taking to heart those of his family and friends. Advice and wish-you-wells out of his own deep pockets were always available when the time was right or the mood struck. "I think dying feels soft, like feathers tickling your nose," he told me, not long before his transplant. In the plane, flying home, I tried to focus on those words, like open air, an open thought left drifting for me to catch hold of. Had Micah known, even then?

I gripped Micah's backpack while his body rode below me in the belly of the plane. My feet touched the cabin floor, but I felt as if I was floating above it. Around me, I could hear muddled conversations, but no real words. My mind worked in slow motion, casting spells on the voice of the flight attendant who offered me coffee or juice, the captain announcing our arrival in San Francisco. I departed the plane but stood on the gangplank, not wanting to leave my son's body to strangers, to the baggage handlers responsible for lifting it, placing it in the hearse that was waiting to take him home to Sonora. I saw my sisters, Jan and Carol, my friend Jan Lekas, waiting in the terminal. They hugged me when I walked down the ramp, sobbing, supporting as best they could. Jan Lekas left after we gathered my luggage, would see me in a couple of days, she said, at Micah's service. Funeral and service were disassociated concepts. I nodded my head, telling her, yes, I'll see you then, but did not associate the word 'service', the process, the act, a funeral, to Micah.

The car ride home was long. The highway seemed endless, a long black strip of asphalt heading forward, but getting nowhere. Driving with my sisters, there was nothing to hold me back: the illness, the pokes and prods, the harsh lights and stale air, the doctors and nurses coming and going, the despair, the inhumanity -- the whole nightmare -- I let it all go in a deluge of tears.

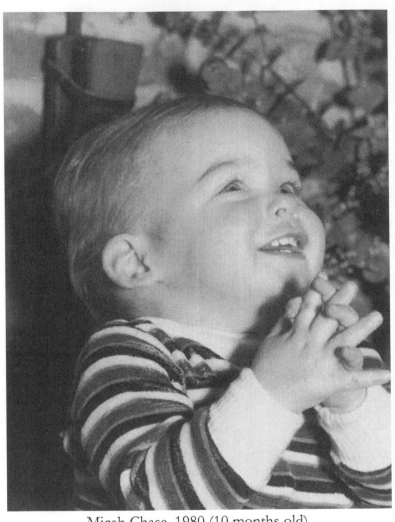

Micah Chase, 1980 (10 months old)

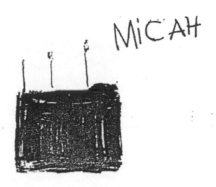

MICAH

"I love birthday cakes and my family. If I had all the money in the world, this is what I would do: I would give my mom some flowers. I would give my brother a toy truck. I would give my dad a bike. I would give my cousin Kippy a really big fish."

by Micah Chase age 5, 1984

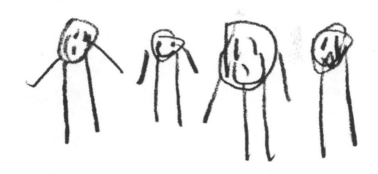

157

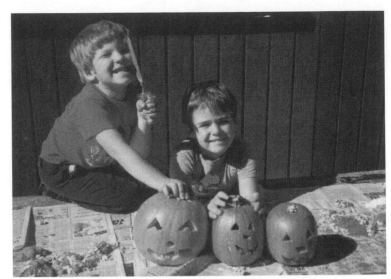

Micah and Nick at home on Big Hill

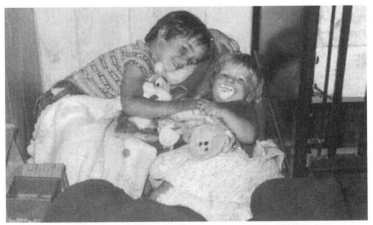

Micah and Nick snuggling in their bedroom

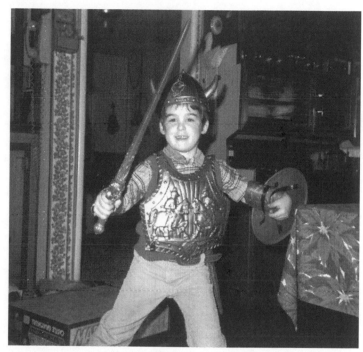

Micah, Christmas 1986

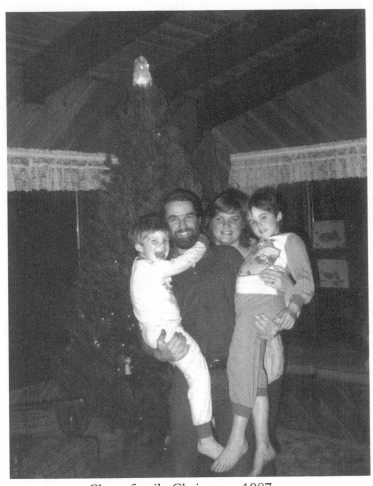

Chase family Christmas, 1987

Dogs
by Micah Chase, 1986
(9 years old)

"I love dogs. My first dogs were Apple and Rock Bottom. Apple was always happy and wagging his tail and Rock Bottom ran on three legs because the other one got hurt when he was a puppy. Rock Bottom was pretty funny because he would chase after rocks when I threw them over the side of the hill.

Now I have a hound dog named Amos. My dad says never to let my mom go in a feed store in the springtime because she loves baby animals and will come home with chickens or ducks or a kitten or a puppy. That's how we got Amos. Nick and me take after Mom and that means trouble for Dad. As soon as the three of us saw that little red hound dog in a box that said FREE on the side of the road, with his long floppy ears and his big droopy eyes we all went "Awww," and then we went "Oooo" and that was it!

That is how we got Amos.

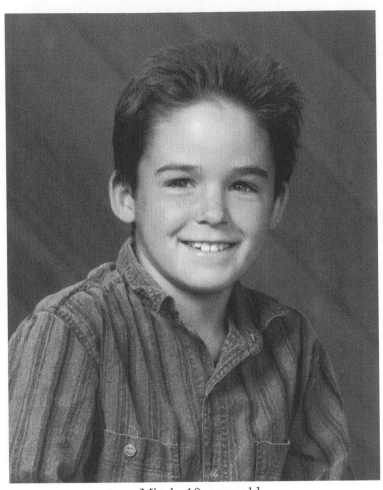
Micah, 10 years old

M arvelous

I ncredible

C reative

A wesome

H appy

C ool

H ip

A ttentive

S tudly

E ducational

163

Rules You Must Follow In My House
by Micah Chase, age 10

1. Never turn the channel on the T.V. when my dad is watching the baseball game or he will wrinkle up his eyebrows at you.

2. Always say good things about my mom's cooking.

3. Never hit or punch my little brother or you will be sent home.

4. Always say please and thank you or mom and dad will think you are rude.

6. Never go in my room without permission or you will get mauled.

7. When you're done going to the bathroom always clean the pee off the seat.

8. Always keep my room clean or else you will have to clean it up totally!

9. Always brush your teeth or you will have to go to the dentist.

10. Never yell from a distance or you will get a lecture.

11. You must know how to play baseball and climb trees.

12. You must love dogs and animals of all kinds.

13. Mostly though, you must always have fun!

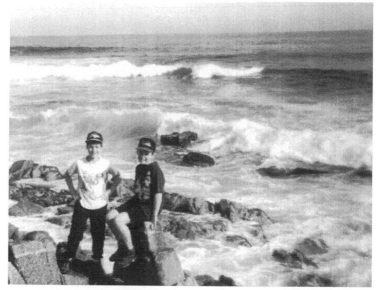

Micah and Nick in Monterey, summer 1992

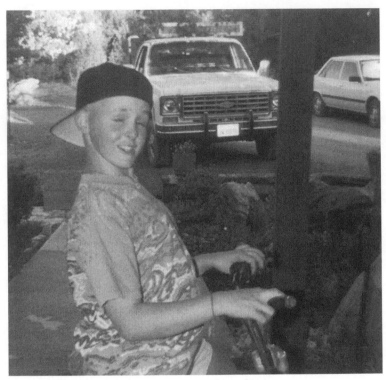

Micah, home after chemo

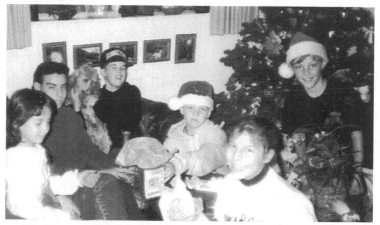

Christmas, 1992 – The big gift – a trip to Hawaii
From left: Season, Kip, Butchy, Micah, Nick,
Katy, and Levi

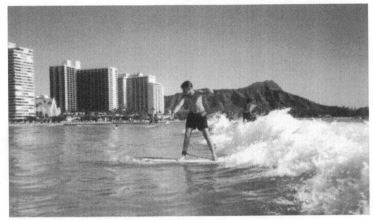

Micah surfing on Waikiki Beach, 1993

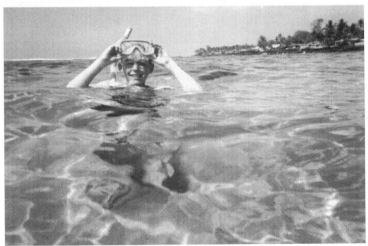

Micah snorkling

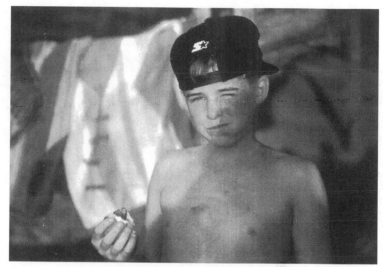

Micah in Hawaii, 1993 (14 years old)

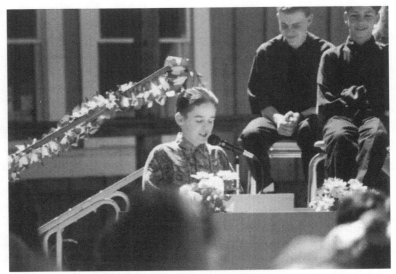

Micah giving his eighth grade graduation speech.

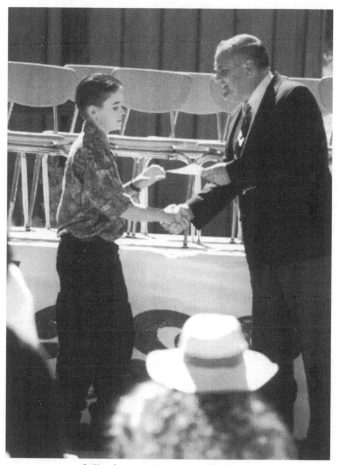

Micah receiving his diploma.

Chapter 14

Over those next few days, my body felt as if it were filled with tiny bouncing balls of electricity, statically charged, trapped in a vortex. People were talking, offering Kleenex, rubbing my shoulders, telling me to eat, to sleep, to talk if it helped. I could see them and hear them, but they existed in the shadows of a past life; in that moment, in the present, my only perception was of a gaping hole, cut ragged and haphazard in the center of my world.

As Micah's family, we each chose our own way in those first, long hours. We went through the motions of surviving, of doing the things we had to do -- breathing because we had no choice, existing in a place where we no longer had any control. It is difficult to figure out what to do with your life when you have suffered such a loss, but that was our chore: Del and me, Nick, grandmas and grandpas, aunts and uncles, cousins, friends. People cooked and brought food to the house, washed our dishes, vacuumed my floors. They brought flowers, potted plants, and sympathy cards. Someone started a journal of thoughts and feelings about Micah. As friends came and went, they added to the book, sharing fun times, adventures, and misadventures. I heard for the first time about some 'near misses' Micah and his friends had while riding their bikes on the ditch trail near our house, climbing into a large water pipe and sailing through it downhill into a pond they were forbidden to play in. I looked into the faces of Jason, Brian, Aaron, Jenny, Mindy, Christina, Austin, and Sarah, realizing they carried with them bits and pieces of Micah, alive and well, still healthy and whole. In a daze, I read each of their entries in the journal, reining in my desperation by absorbing their words.

In the evenings when things were quiet, I poured through Micah's diary, obsessed at the thought of connecting to pieces of him I might have missed along the way. I poured through his pictures and found stories long forgotten. In his suitcase, still packed from the hospital, alongside a book of crossword puzzles and a May 1992 issue of the Beckett Baseball Card Price Guide, I found the last story he had written while in Oakland Children's Hospital:

By Micah
Oakland Children's Hospital, June 1992

"I have a lot of time to think when I'm in the hospital. Right now I'm sitting on my bed and I can see a little girl with curly blonde hair and big blue eyes standing with her IV pole just outside her room. I think she's about six years old. Maurice told me she has AIDS. She's watching the nurses right now and she looks really sad. I wonder if she ever thinks about why she got sick, like I do. Maybe she's too young to understand. Maurice has bone cancer in his leg. He's supposed to walk with crutches but sometimes he doesn't. Nurse Debbie told me to get after him if he comes in here without his crutches. She said he might have to get his leg amputated if he's not really careful. Maurice lives with his grandma in Nevada. He says his mother is on drugs and she can't take care of him very well. He really

173

loves my mom and wishes his mom was like her.

"Maurice didn't have a choice about who his parents were or how they would treat him once he was born. There are angels here, in this hospital. I hear the nurses talking about them all the time. "Little angels, every one," they say. Maurice is African American. I am a mix of a lot of things, but mostly I'm Austrian, English, Irish, and a little Choctaw Indian. There's an Asian kid, down the hall with a brain tumor, and there's a Mexican kid with Hodgkin's Lymphoma. My mom told me a story about angels once. She said they watch over all of us. It doesn't matter who we are or what color of skin we have.

"One time, with my family in Yosemite, I saw a bald eagle. I've always loved eagles. I like the way they glide in the sky and how they watch over the land. They remind me of angels because of that. I think about eagle feathers being sacred to the Native Americans and angel wings being sacred to people who are Christian.

"I have a lot of time to think right now, and I wonder why people think they are so different from each other. I am in this hospital with kids who may look different than me but we are all really the same. None of us can help where we were born or who our parents are.

Here in the hospital we're all just kids. Eagles fly with the angels here. I wish that was true everywhere.

"When I grow up, I'm going to be a doctor. I'm going to invent things that make sick kids well and make their time in the hospital hurt less and be easier. I'm going to teach people that we're all one big family and should always act that way."

Holding this last story Micah had written to my chest, I called out to him, wishing him to defy death and come back to me, half believing he could do it, would walk in the door and say, "Oh, Mom, look at you, all teary and everything. You're being silly!" When he and Nick were little, they

174

once brought me an empty coke bottle, claiming that if I filled it with my tears, and if tears were worth money, we would be rich. "We could sell this at the flea market!" Micah teased as Nick giggled along. It was true; I cried easily over old movies, sad stories, other people's misfortunes. Only now, it was Micah I cried over, and his silliness and shenanigans could no longer stop the flow, make me laugh or play or feel normal. Normal. The words bit at my ears.

Three days at home, and I had not heard from Del. He was still on the road, and I could only imagine how hard it was for him to drive alone with his grief, across state borders and into the unfamiliar territory that waited for him. We needed to talk. There was so much to say, so many decisions to make; the funeral director was waiting for direction regarding Micah's burial, his service. Upon request, my sister Jan, Uncle John, and I met with him at the funeral parlor to discuss the different options. Warning me before hand that it would be difficult, he escorted me to a room full of boxes, coffins made of bronze, gold, and silver. Some were inscribed, some had pictures of trees, one had an etching of Yosemite's Half Dome across the side.

This couldn't be real. This couldn't be happening. I felt lightheaded and reached for Jan. Micah was supposed to be starting high school with his friends. In the stack of mail on the table at home were his high school transcripts. He had gotten all the classes he signed up for before we left for Texas: Physical education, English 1, Beginning Wood Shop, Algebra 1, Life Skills, Keyboarding. He had a student number: 3546. He had a locker. Jason, Jenny, Mindy and Christina, Sarah, Austin, Jonathon, Aaron, Tony, they were

175

all registered at Sonora High. As at Belleview, they would be going through school together, a team, a group of friends who had been there for each other since they were small. Micah should be there! This wasn't right! It wasn't fair! *I love you, Micah! I'm sorry! I'm so, so sorry!*

I gathered brochures, pictures of different styles of caskets to show Del, trying just to keep breathing while deciding on the best choice for Micah. In the end, we kept it simple, like the land, like the Big Hill where he grew up, like the house we had built by hand as a family. The coffin we chose was made of etched red cedar, draped inside with white satin and with a white satin pillow as a headrest. Micah loved the smell of cedar, had lived around the tree, the wood, all his life. He had been carving small floating boats, gnomes, animals, and crude tools since he was big enough to safely hold a whittling knife. And the pillow would make him happy, I thought. Its shiny softness reminded me of his baby blanket, his 'silky', he called it. He had slept with that blanket, carried it with him until his years of loving it wore the satin away.

Del made it home in the afternoon of the fourth day. He drove into our yard and into the midst of planning Micah's service. Soon we were talking about where, when, and how we would like the ceremony performed. Ceremony, to me, had become the optimal word; the service would be a ceremony of Micah's life. His friends had suffered yet another loss over the summer; a student in their class had died in an automobile accident and the funeral had been hard on them. Some were frightened by the words, the warnings of the minister who spoke. We listened to their thoughts and wishes, as Micah would have

176

listened. We decided to have the service outdoors, at the cemetery, a combination of a Christian ceremony and a Native American blessing, officiated by our pastor friend, Jerome, and Jesse, a Native American Spiritual Leader.

That day, we stood in a circle and were blessed by their prayers and by the burning essences of sage and cedar. Two friends played their guitars and sang *The Dance,* by Garth Brooks and *Tears in Heaven,* by Eric Clapton. People shared stories about Micah. Nick passed out little cards with the picture of a pine tree, a cloud, and an eagle in flight on the cover. Inside was Micah's celebration of life announcement, the date of his birth and the date of his death.

I must have repeated Micah's story a hundred times, to family and friends, acquaintances at his funeral, and later, on the phone, in the grocery store, at the post office. Telling and retelling a story makes it real, and I suppose that's what I needed to have happen. As is typical of those in grief, Nick and I found peace in hidden meanings -- sightings of clouds that were particularly beautiful, a heart-shaped stone newly discovered, a golden sunset reminiscent of those in Hawaii, a favorite song of Micah's played on the radio as we were talking about him. We were often melancholy, but always, when thinking of or talking about Micah, a smile crossed our faces, his zest for life still as contagious as ever.

For the loved ones left behind, life becomes a series of firsts: the first day back to work for Del and me, the first day of school for Nick. Nick and I held our breath as we climbed out of the car, trying to remember how Micah had done it after his bone marrow biopsies, standing tall and erect, walking proudly, with a smile on his face and a look of confidence in his eyes. Nick's teacher told me afterward how heroic he was that morning, how he stood in front of his 6th grade class and announced Micah's death. "If you have anything you want to know, ask me," he told them. "I don't want anyone saying anything that's not true about my brother, so if there's something you want to know, ask me, instead of someone else." It was typical of my boys to defend each other to the end. As brothers, they would argue about little things (who got to sit in the front seat of the car, who got to pick out the ice cream when we went grocery shopping, who got the autographed baseball card from a Giants game in San Francisco) but when it came to big things, like honor and respect, they never faltered in their concern for each other's feelings.

That winter was full of firsts: setting the table with three plates instead of four, kissing one child goodnight, instead of two; figuring out how to get up in the morning, to sleep at night, to function in a way that seemed normal. Sitting on Micah's bed one day, I mourned over his clothes, his shoes, his toys. Boxing things up seemed too final. It meant he wasn't coming home, that he wasn't just down the road at Jason's house and wouldn't be bounding in the door after awhile with an adventure to share, a story to tell, a new song to play on his stereo. I couldn't decide what to keep, what not to keep, what should go to Nick, Micah's cousins, his friends. As was typical, in the end, the kids helped me decide. After Nick made his choices and those things were set aside, I invited his cousins in and then his friends. They each were respectful, picking something to remember Micah by, a tangible gift to keep forever. A favorite hat. A baseball card. A special shirt or CD. When the giving, the sharing, was done, and I was alone again in Micah's room, I cried. There was so much more. Micah's life was in his room, all the things he had collected in his fourteen years: his geode collection, his baseball card collection, favorite baseball caps, his favorite music -- his t-shirt with a picture of Bugs Bunny in sagging pants, both on the front, and on the back. The smell of him still lingered on his clothes. In the closet were his favorite tennis shoes, laced up in that funny way. His drawings, his journals, his life was in his room. Out of utter despair, I decided to leave things as they were until some necessity demanded otherwise.

Chapter 15

One night in September, I sat on the floor in our living room beside a large cardboard file box; spread across the floor were bills, letters, and affidavits. They had been accumulating steadily since before we had come home from Texas. Our total debt owed to Ketchell Hospital, including the bone marrow transplant, the time Micah spent in intensive care, and charges for his after-care had swelled to $270,000.00. As each bill arrived, I remained numb to their meaning, setting them aside until the stack was too big to ignore. Where was Micah in the midst of all of those pages, his eyes, his hair, his smile?

Del looked past me with blind eyes, away from the boxes, away from the memories. I asked him for help. "Okay," he said, but turned instead to the remote control, a baseball game he was watching on television. I opened my mouth to ask him again but didn't, recognizing his avoidance, understanding it in a weird, *wish-I-could-go-there*, way.

Nick was lying next to me doing his homework. His stack of papers was shorter than mine, and he kept glancing over as if he wished he could do something to help. I patted his leg, feeling sure that he needed comforting as much as I did. As I touched his calf, I realized my fingers were numb. I'd been clinching my fists so tightly the palms of my hands were white, looking as pale as Micah looked before a blood transfusion. My eyes shifted to the black water stain that had been growing on the cedar paneled wall opposite the bathroom. We'd developed a leaky pipe, and neither Del nor I could verify for the plumber how long the problem had existed. The damage was serious, however, and in his effort to find the cause, the plumber discovered a termite infestation in the substructure of the house. I turned away from the tarnished wainscoting, closing my eyes to the beginning of our broken home. What had once seemed like a firm foundation was now crumbling beneath my feet, and there was nothing to do but give my attention to Nick and the unpaid stack of hospital bills.

Nick was struggling with his algebra. His brow furrowed as he brushed eraser crumbs from his worksheet, fumbling for the answer to some illusive equation. He was so sweet, so caring, so innocent -- too young to have to deal with the death of his older brother. School had always been a priority in our house; homework was done without protest, a component of family time -- me beside the boys at the dining room table or on the living room floor, cooking dinner or reading, but ready to offer my help if needed, Micah answering Nick's questions when a new concept required some explaining. Where were we going to find the money to help Nick with his college education when the time came? The kids' college fund was in its infancy when we depleted it in favor of staying afloat, meeting the demands of our ever growing dependency on hospitals and critical medical care. The stack of blue paper at my side was two inches thick, too heavy to ignore, each page with Micah's name on it. Micah Charles Chase, my child, my responsibility, his debt, my debt, his heart beating through the palm of my hand as I lifted the stack and laid it on my lap. Through all of our twenty-year marriage, Del and I had never been late in paying our house payment, our utility bills, various other small debts. We lived pay-check to pay-check but we managed. We had good credit. Two years earlier, we'd had a small savings. I was fretting over the thought of an empty bank account when the phone rang.

Somehow, between the social workers in Texas and in California, I had been put in touch with the Volunteer Legal Services Project and had been assigned a volunteer attorney. He introduced himself when I answered the phone and asked about the basics of our situation, about Micah's procedure, the insurance company's denial, the amount we owed Ketchell Hospital. His advice was not very encouraging. It was tough to take on a major insurance company, he said. At this point, it would be nearly impossible to recoup any monies from them. He could write a letter to Ketchell Hospital on our behalf, explaining our financial situation, stating that paying their bill at this time would require the sale of our home, but his best hope in that regard was simply to buy us some time. My mind wandered as he talked, and I thought about selling the house we had built by hand. I imagined being homeless, wandering the streets of Sonora with no home to go home to. I glanced at the blackened wall again, wondering if we could even put the house up for sale now that it was damaged, making a mental note to call a real estate agent and educate myself, and then I struggled to refocus on the conversation at hand. As far as the letters to Ketchell Hospital, I told the attorney that I had sent several myself in hopes of delaying payment but had no luck and no response other than receiving more bills. He assured me that he would try again. Memories of the anguish in Micah's face the day we learned of the insurance company denying payment of his bone marrow transplant caused a swell of angry spasms in the pit of my stomach. The thought of Ketchell Hospital delaying his critical treatment because they had not yet been assured payment caused tears to pool in my eyes and Nick to snuggle closer, understanding without words.

Two weeks earlier, during a broadcast from our local radio station, I heard that John Garamendi, the Insurance Commissioner for the State of California was going to be in Sonora. I went to speak with him about Micah's situation, the problem of insurance companies refusing to pay for doctor prescribed medical treatments. The venue was in a local breakfast house, and it was noisy and crowded when I arrived. Mr. Garamendi was gracious and gave me some time, but it was difficult to have much of a conversation. Though he was sympathetic to my cause, he emphasized that it would be nearly impossible to prove the insurance company wrong, that I was fighting a difficult battle. Kelly George, Micah's doctor from Sonora, tried once again to intercede on our behalf. He wrote Mr. Garamendi a follow up letter and included a letter of support that he had received from Dr. Klu:

September 30, 1993
Dear Commissioner Garamendi:

I would like to bring to your attention a patient of mine who recently died from cancer. His name was Micah. Over the last two to three months, Micah had been in and out of remission from his chemotherapy but showed a slow but steady worsening of his condition. It had been made clear from the beginning of his care with the cancer experts at Children's Hospital in Oakland and at U.C.S.F. that he was going to need a bone marrow transplant if he wished to have any hope of survival. During this time period his insurance company had been supporting Micah as he had full coverage under their benefits package. They were aware from the early start that bone marrow transplantation was something that was definitely needed in his case and never showed any signs of denying his care during this early period of time.

However, as his case became worse and it became more apparent that he would need care outside of the State, the insurance company started balking at its responsibility regarding his care. Once an institution in Texas was found that could do the bone marrow transplant the insurance company was very slow to address our concerns regarding whether insurance would pay this or not and eventually decided to deny it. First saying that the bone marrow transplant could be done in the State of California as their main reason for denial and finally saying that because it was an "experimental" form of therapy that they would not cover it. Nevertheless, the parents, feeling that this was their last hope did take Micah to Ketchell Hospital in Houston, Texas where bone marrow transplantation was done, but unfortunately it wasn't successful and Micah died.

Commissioner, I would appreciate any help you or your office staff could give us in trying to get this insurance company to essentially fulfill its obligation to the Chase family. As things stand now, the Chase family is in debt to a great degree for the bone marrow transplantation done in Houston and the very real possibility of them losing their home and other worldly possessions to pay off this debt. I am forwarding with this letter, other letters from other health care professionals at Children's Hospital in Oakland, from Dr. Klu at Ketchell Hospital in Houston, and from the transplant team at the University of California, San Francisco Bone Marrow Transplant Center that substantiates my argument in this behalf.

Sincerely,
Kelly George, M.D.

Letter addressed to Dr. George from Dr. Klu
September 29, 1993

I am writing to further discuss the use of mismatched marrow transplantation for the treatment of leukemia. As less than 30% of leukemia patients requiring bone marrow transplantation has matched relatives to be used as a donor, it is not surprising that an alternate source of bone marrow cells is required to provide treatment for the majority (over 70%) who might benefit from this procedure. The availability of unrelated marrow donors in the past several years has provided 30-50% of this group of patients with a source of marrow for transplantation but the remainder of patients will have to receive marrow from mismatched family relatives.

The use of mismatched family donors of bone marrow transplantation is not new. A number of trials published in strategic journals have been available since the mid 1980's and I am enclosing a list for your reference. It appears from these reports that mismatched related donors are a legitimate source of bone marrow for poor risk patients whose disease had failed other conventional therapies. Micah was transplanted according to an institution-approved and NCI-reviewed protocol, indicating that his treatment is not performed ad-hoc or on a random basis. Mismatched related donor transplants are being performed in other states including Iowa, Kentucky, South Carolina and New York. I understand that no active protocol was available in California when Micah required his marrow transplant and he was accepted into our program for his treatment.

In summary, an increasing number of patients are receiving marrow transplants from donors other than matched siblings and we are seeing a trend that alternative bone marrow donors provide the answer to the majority of patients who require marrow transplantations at this moment. Thank you once again for discussing Micah's case with me and please do not hesitate to contact me if you have any further questions regarding his management.

Yours sincerely,
Dr. Klu

After reading the statements of Micah's primary doctors, it was difficult to imagine how there could have been a controversy regarding payment of his transplant. Fact after fact was established through their competency and experience. Issue after issue brought up as a reason for denial by the insurance company was addressed and substantiated. My frustration grew stronger as each letter brought Micah's rights into question, as a patient, a human being, a child suffering from cancer. Grieving him was difficult enough; suffering the atrocity of abuse within the medical system I had trusted with my son's life was like being trapped inside a cement mixer, crushed and tossed about with little hope of escape.

Lying on the floor next to the hospital bills, copies of the letters from Micah's doctors, and the attorney from Volunteer Legal Services, was a letter I'd recently received from the KCRA Channel 3 news studio in Sacramento. I picked it up, and reread it, unable to believe that I had been invited to attend a town hall meeting in Sacramento on October 3rd. Should I accept the invitation, I would meet President Bill Clinton and ask him a question of my choice about health care reform.

I discussed the invitation with Terri Dixon, a friend and teacher at Belleview School. She was diagnosed with

187

multiple sclerosis just months after Micah's diagnosis of leukemia and had experienced problems with nonpayment of insurance claims for medications prescribed by her doctor. After talking about the town hall meeting, she told me a story about an incident that happened on the playground a year earlier. "I slipped and fell down," she said. "I was scared and embarrassed, but before I had time to think, there was Micah. We shared a moment," she told me, "one that I'll never forget. He looked right into my eyes, and I saw his compassion. I knew that he understood exactly how I felt. He helped me up and into my classroom, smiled that unforgettable smile of his and gave me a hug, then went on about his business. Micah kept my fall private, just between him and me, and that meant a great deal at the time. He was an exceptional kid," she said. "You go to that meeting for Micah *and* for me. Sharing a story can bring about necessary change. Sometimes, you have to go public with private issues."

Deciding to go before a national audience to make public Micah's personal struggle was not easy. He had agreed to interviews with newspaper reporters for his bone marrow drives, but getting him to do them took a lot of convincing. In some of the pictures taken at that time, it was easy to see the hesitation in his eyes. The leukemia had been his battle from the start; he wanted no sympathy, no special acknowledgement of his disease. I tried to rationalize the differences in time and place, to put myself in Micah's shoes. It was easy to picture his frustration, to remember the effects of delay after delay, denial after denial. All of Micah's life, he had been a great debater; he argued for what he believed in with full conviction. It angered him when he felt someone had been judged unfairly or that an issue was decided upon without listening to the facts. We'd had wonderful discussions about relationships between people, their cultures, geography, religions, and the effect of those things on the way we live our lives. We had talked a lot about prejudice. He'd experienced it himself on a minor level. In the third grade, he had a long-term substitute teacher who was good-natured with the girls in the class but could be harsh and sometimes cruel to the boys. In the fourth grade, he entered a bicycle race and won but was accused of miscounting his laps because the person officiating felt he could not have possibly rounded the track more times on his little Schwinn Predator than another boy who had ridden a brand new twelve-speed mountain bike. I had watched the whole race from the playground where I was doing yard duty. I'd counted Micah's laps and knew he had rightfully won.

Micah knew that prejudice takes many forms and understood it to be unjust, whether by judgment or opinion without full examination of the facts or irrational suspicion or hatred of a particular group, race, or religion. The denial of payment for his bone marrow transplant was prejudice on another level. The judgment of a major corporation took away his rights, caused unnecessary pain and suffering by their preconceived, unfavorable convictions. Micah was a fighter as far as his illness was concerned. He never gave up. He went on about his business, standing strong, walking with his head up, determined and proud. Hoping for an assist to help Micah score the point of his life became my focus as I scribbled version after version of the *one perfect question* I would ask the President of the United States.

Grammar had nothing to do with it. Neither did perfect spelling. It was all about the truth of right and wrong as my parents had taught me and as I had taught Micah. It was about the desperate look on his face, the confusion in his eyes, when he realized that his life, as far as our insurance company was concerned, came down to an issue of dollars and cents.

Chapter 16

The KCRA producers graciously allowed a support person to come with me to the studio, understanding that I was still very emotional so soon after Micah's death. Del was not interested in going, and Nick was too young according to the studio representative, so I asked my sister Jan to go. She drove, concentrating on the road as we dropped three thousand feet from the foothills of the Sierra Nevada into the Sacramento Valley through a patchwork of farmland, along ribbons of gray asphalt hemmed with housing tracts, strip malls, the outskirts of Sacramento. She steered her truck to the left and then the right, calm but pressing ahead, her back stiff, leaning forward with the flow of traffic, urging other drivers on.

Through the corner of my eye, I could see cars passing by, people going to work, shopping, picking their kids up from school -- people carrying on with their daily lives as if nothing was different, as if everything was fine. I gripped with both hands the index card on which I'd written my question and the statement I'd prepared for my five minutes of air-time, the five-minutes I had been granted to speak with President Clinton.

"We're here," Jan said. "You ready?"

I took a deep breath and nodded yes.

The air around me mutated, felt corrosive, and cold. I shuddered and closed my eyes, feeling lost and confused, wondering how I had got from my quiet life on a mountain top to an invitation-only visit with the President of the United States.

Your child is not supposed to die first! A mother is not supposed to outlive her children!

Dream-like images filtered in and out, distilling my fear, engaging my anger. The words on Micah's burial stone ran through my mind: *We'll love you forever. Son. Brother. Friend.* Bruises, black and purple, bounced before my eyes, memories of a happy, active boy turned quiet and moody -- a battery of tests and the deadly diagnosis that tumbled from the lips of strangers: Acute Myelocytic Leukemia. I thought about the hospitals, the lights and stale air, the doctors and nurses, coming and going. I focused on the insurance company's denial of Micah's bone marrow transplant.

I read aloud the instructions on where to park. The lot was cordoned off with large barricades, ropes, and police tape. A single tour bus sat like a shiny metal sentinel at the far right end, secure, but a little bit menacing. Jan parked the truck, and we got out and walked toward the bus, toward a metal detector, secret servicemen, Sacramento police with dogs on leashes. The German Shepherds sniffed up, down, in trees, around manholes. I handed a police officer my invitation, and the dogs sniffed me too. They sniffed Jan. We were told to walk through the metal detector. Too nervous to speak, I nodded and did as instructed.

I opened and closed my mouth, checking, hoping it

would cooperate when the time came. I picked my way through tiers of emotions, praying that I would be able to speak my mind about the injustices Micah suffered, the prejudice on a corporate level imposed at a time when no person should have to endure such cruelty. I reread the statement I had written, erasing parts, the ashes of my words falling fruitlessly at my feet. I fumbled for new words, knowing there were no right words, wondering how I could express the pain I felt, the anguish, in only five minutes. Again, I tumbled backwards in my recollection of events: *"Your insurance company is refusing to pay for Micah's transplant. We've tried everything, written letters, held conference calls.* And the final insult from an insurance company doctor: *"This boy is going to die anyway. Why should we put that kind of money out?"*

A representative of the studio took a quick glance at my index card and told me that my statement was too long. "The question needs to be shorter," she said. I held the index card to my chest, took a breath, and started over. Jan and I and forty-eight other people were escorted into the bus. I wrote while we drove several blocks to the KCRA studio. *Tiny white pills, larger orange ones, and an IV drip set to run over a course of five days. Micah's counts dropped quickly; isolation rules were put into effect -- masks, gloves, no physical contact with bare hands.*

We sat on the bus while the dogs went to work again, checking everything: the bus, the grounds, the entry to the studio. The door opened and secret servicemen poured in, walking up and down the aisles, checking overhead, under our seats, seeing through eyes trained to look beyond the parameters of normal vision.

193

Dear God, I prayed. *Help me be strong. Keep me upright.* I glanced at my sister. I thanked God for her, for my family, and friends, their love and support. *At night, I lay watching my son -- so quiet, so still. Nothing passed by me, not an involuntary jerk of an arm or attempt to roll over. I saw every breath, heard every whimper, each interruption, every nurse entering the room to administer medication or draw Micah's blood or check his pumps -- four of them beeping simultaneously into the night.*

An unfamiliar voice called me back to the present. "You'll be the first person to speak," I was told.

My knees buckled. I reached for my sister's hand as we exited the bus. We walked across the parking lot, through yet another metal detector and into the studio. The forum was laid out in a semi-circle. We were escorted to a seat in the front near a red-carpeted, circular stage, a raised area twenty feet around. Secret service men were clustered together, cautious, eyes scanning the growing assembly of people.

When everyone was seated, the doors behind us were locked. A newscaster, someone familiar, entered the room and took a microphone. "Ladies and gentlemen, we thank you for coming to this first in a series of Town Hall Meetings," Stan Atkinson said. "It is my honor this afternoon to introduce our distinguished guest, President Bill Clinton.

President Clinton entered the room, tall, proud, smiling, waving. We stood and applauded. He nodded, graciously. Jan squeezed my hand, acknowledging my fear.

"Mr. President, your first question comes from a woman from Sonora, California."

Somehow I stood, walked down two stairs, to the

194

podium.

"Mr. President," I stumbled. "I'm here for my son, because of my son, Micah. I lost him four weeks ago, to leukemia."

"I'm sorry," President Clinton said. "I'm truly sorry for your loss."

"Our insurance company refused to pay for the bone marrow transplant recommended by my son's doctors. Their delays and eventual denial was valuable time lost, and while we waited, Micah's condition weakened beyond the point he could endure the rigors of the transplant he eventually received. Their treatment of him was cruel and unconscionable. Micah's rights as a medical patient and human being were violated horribly. I want to ask you about health care reform, Mr. President. I want to talk to you about the misuse of power by insurance companies in this country and their growing tendency toward denial of doctor recommended forms of treatment for their patients."

Jan wrote as President Clinton spoke, documenting the portions of his response I missed due to the pounding of my heart: His plan would cover certain conditions like leukemia. It would cover the best available treatments recommended by doctors. "However, there has to be evidence that the treatment might work, so in the case of a bone marrow transplant, where there is evidence that it often has been effective, the plan should cover that," he said. "And that's the way we tried to set it up. In other words, to be less restrictive than most insurance policies are today, but still leave doctors with their considered medical judgment, some ground not to do things that don't make any sense at all."

195

President Clinton spoke for several minutes before the KCRA newscaster urged him on to the next person, the next question that needed answering. I walked back to my seat, sat down and bit my lip to quiet my nerves. *I took a deep breath, hesitating no longer than a moment to search the doctor's face once more, before words came out of my mouth I never imagined I'd say. "Then no. No more tubes, no more pumps. No catheters or shots. Can you make him comfortable?"*

"Excuse me just a minute," the President said. He broke away from the newscaster and turned back to me. "Please, I'm not done talking with this woman."

I stood, unsure what to say, or do.

"First, I want to thank you for coming here today," he said. "I want to tell you how humbled I feel. It must take an awful lot of courage for her to come here within a month of losing her child," he said to the newscaster, the audience. "I thank her."

Everyone in the audience stood and clapped.

Eighteen questions followed mine, and when the Town Hall Meeting ended, Jan and I were invited into a reception line to meet the President and speak with him again. "Thank you for acknowledging our need for health care reform," I said, as I shook his hand. "I support what you are doing and wish you the best."

"I wish there was something more I could do," he told me. "My thoughts will be with you and your family."

Driving home from Sacramento, Jan and I laughed about silly things, anything. We shared memories about our trip to Hawaii. I talked about snorkeling with Nick, when he and I went out farther in the ocean than I realized, how I

196

had heard an alarm of some sort, a loud horn, and panicked, imagining it was a shark alert. I pulled Nick through the water like a mad woman, trying to save him from a nonexistent threat. "Mom!" he said, between gulps of water. "You're drowning me, Mom! Stop!"

My sisters and I were good at listening to our kids. It was something we learned from our parents. My mother had always been there for each of us over the years, listening, counseling, gently reprimanding, but never judging. After Micah's death, I tried to answer Nick's questions honestly but keep the stress of financial concerns as far from his daily life as possible. He joined a football team, saw his friends, did okay in school, other than a problem with talking too much in class. Talking had always been an issue for Nick, but now, with everything we'd gone through, it became a necessity. "When I talk," he told me, "I don't think about things as much." It was something I understood well, but his teacher at school didn't get it, so he spent a lot of time in the hall for being disruptive in class. Watching his transition from being a brother to an only child was as difficult as my own. I didn't recognize myself in the mirror anymore. My name was still Shelley Chase, and I was still Del's wife, the mother of Micah and Nick, but that's where things had changed in a way that was difficult to explain. I heard Nick fumble for words when someone asked him questions about his family. I fumbled for words when someone asked me how many children I had. "I have two, well, I had two. I have one now. My older son passed away."

When Micah was ill, and his counts were low, he would wear his mask when we went grocery shopping. Mothers would guide their children to the other side of the aisle when they saw him, to avoid any possible contact, contamination. As the weeks passed, after Micah's death, I saw the same thing happen but for different reasons. On the street one day, I saw a woman I knew. I waved and walked toward her, but she put her head down and turned away. Avoidance and denial are sometimes easier than confrontation, I learned. I don't know what I would have done without the support of those I loved. It's a necessary part of recovery, having people around to listen when you tell the same story for the hundredth time, to cry with you, and make you laugh. My friend, Terry Gonzales, would stick her fingers in her ears and make funny faces if she saw that I was having a hard time at work. She would turn my tears into laugher with a silly story or a cock-eyed grin. Nick was lucky in that way. His friends, like Micah's, had been lifelong and were there to help him keep some normalcy in his life.

Normalcy within grief is a hard thing to come by though, and with hospital bills arriving at regular intervals, the idea of finding some healing time and resolution was never a convenience allowed us. My files grew thicker. The phone bill grew larger at the end of each month. Still, we tried to maintain. Del spent more time in his garage, working on projects, puttering with his CB radio equipment. After helping Nick with his homework at night, after he'd gone to bed, I wrote letters, made notes about articles I read from books, journals, anything substantial that offered advice or provided a way to focus my thoughts.

After speaking with President Clinton in Sacramento, I sent him a thank you letter, along with a picture of Micah. I also sent a letter to Hillary Clinton, hoping for some further information about her proposed health care reform. A month later, I received a letter from the President, thanking me and again offering his condolences.

November 3, 1993

Mr. and Mrs. Del Chase

Dear Shelley and Del:

Hillary and I were sorry to learn of
the death of your son Micah. We hope that
the love and support of your family and
friends will sustain and comfort you during
this difficult time.

The photograph you sent will help me
keep your son in mind as I work to reform our
nation's health care system.

You and Nick are in our thoughts and
prayers.

Sincerely,

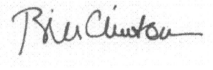

Touched by the President's consideration for my feelings, and by the fact that he listened to our story and cared about what had happened to Micah, Nick sent a follow-up letter, a thank you note to the White House. Again, to my amazement, we received a response.

THE WHITE HOUSE

WASHINGTON

November 30, 1993

Nick Chase

Dear Nick:

　　Thank you for writing me to let me know how your family has been since I spoke with your mother in Sacramento.

　　I'm sorry that you have had to go through such a difficult time. You and your parents are in my thoughts and prayers.

Sincerely,

Bill Clinton

I believe that President Clinton's letter helped Nick cope. This simple acknowledgement of Nick's feelings, the fact that someone as important as the President of the United States cared, meant a great deal. Many times within the hospital setting, I saw the siblings of the kids in treatment come to visit. I saw the way they existed on the outside looking in, concerned, scared, even jealous on occasion. At times, I saw resentment in their eyes. I also saw tremendous love and support. One day, I heard the sister of a young boy who had hemophilia crying in the hallway just outside Micah's room. I invited her in to talk, and she came willingly, needing desperately to connect with someone she thought might understand. I could see the turmoil going on in her brother's room, the parents at his bedside, the rush of nurses taking vitals, trying to assess his condition. Tina could not have been more than ten years old, but her face, her eyes, showed an emotional toll much greater than that age should have displayed. "I feel guilty," she shared, "for hating my brother today." She should have been at her best friend's birthday party, she told me, but instead, she was in the hospital with Jonah. Again. He had gotten sick, and her parents rushed him to Oakland Children's instead of taking her to the party. She told me she had yelled at him, told him she wished he would die. "I didn't mean it," she sobbed. "Oh please, I didn't mean it," she said, looking anxiously out the door and down the hall toward Jonah's room.

"Jonah knows you didn't mean it, Tina," Micah said. "He knows you love him. When things calm down, you can go give him a hug. It'll be okay, I promise."

Siblings become the forgotten element in a situation

such as ours. We remember to ask the parents how things are; we ask the sick child how he's feeling, but how often do we remember to ask the sibling of a sick child how are they are holding up? How often do we say, *I know this is tough on you. I'm proud of you for being so brave. Let me know if there's anything I can do for you, if there's anything you need.* The hospitalization of a brother or sister is traumatic, requiring the shifting of priorities. Siblings are required to stay with family and friends on many occasions. They have to rely on people other than their parents to get them to school, to after-school activities, to help with homework. They keep their feelings inside, not wanting to worry or stress their parents or their sick brother or sister any more than is necessary. Their grieving starts early and happens on many different levels. As I watched Nick move through his days at school, dark circles under his eyes, standing in the hallway repeatedly, I asked the school counselor to step in. She spoke with Nick and assured me that Nick was working through his anxiety about Micah's death in a way that was best for him. I understood that Nick's teachers considered his talking a disruption in their classes, yet I wished they would think to ask him, *How are you? How are you holding up? Is there anything I can do for you or that you need?* I wanted someone to guide us through a passage that was constantly shifting, a family dynamic that had changed despite all efforts to keep things as balanced as possible.

Chapter 17

On November 9, I received a letter from our insurance carrier, a follow up to the letter sent by Dr. George back in September.

Dear Ms. Chase:

The Department of Insurance advised us of your request for assistance regarding a denied precertification and authorization for referral to Ketchell Hospital in Houston.

Dr. Bustoff, Medical Director for the insurance company, requested Ketchell Hospital's detailed protocol for this procedure after receiving the letter from them indicating that bone marrow transplantation is not an experimental form of therapy.

Ketchell Hospital's statement apparently refers to the BMT procedure itself. At issue is not the BMT procedure, but the application under these circumstances to a patient in full relapse and unresponsive to chemotherapy. We do authorize syngeneic and/or HLA matched allogeneic BMT for appropriate candidates with a variety of diseases including leukemia.

Ketchell Hospital's protocol clearly states the treatment is a pilot study for the purpose of researching the incidence of GVHD in BMT recipients receiving a short course of IL-2 in addition to standard immunosuppressive drugs. The second purpose is to determine the toxicity of a short course of rhu IL-2 early after marrow transplantation.

The informed consent form states participants are at high risk for developing GVHD. It also describes the treatment as research and identifies IL-2 as "an investigational agent." Dr. Klu indicated that only four individuals have been treated under this protocol at Ketchell Hospital, none of them children.

When considering the case, Dr. Bustoff discussed the protocol with several BMT hematologists. They concurred that Micah was not a candidate because he was in relapse and because of the lack of an adequately matched marrow donor. Your medical insurance coverage does not extend to research studies. Micah's coverage as a dependent under your group, excludes benefits for experimental/investigative procedures which are not widely accepted as proven and effective. The denial of your claim is upheld.

Sitting on the floor again with my file box beside me, I looked over the stacks of consent forms Del and I had signed for possible bone marrow transplantation at Oakland Children's Hospital and at U.C.S.F. Every one of them clearly stated that the protocol described was experimental, including both the T-cell and the donor match transplants. I thought back to our transplant consultation in San Francisco, to the doctor's explanation of Graft versus Host disease. I remembered him telling me that he would gladly recommend Micah for a T-cell depleted transplant, that he would make sure there was a bed available for him at any time. I also remembered him saying that the transplant in Texas had better promise. "Unfortunately," he had told us, "it's not one we're offering in California at this time."

The doctors at the insurance company must have had different 'experts' than we had. That much was obvious from the letter I had received. Again, I poured through paperwork, recognizing the contradictions in the statements made by the insurance company versus what I knew to be true based on the opinions of the doctors who had assisted in Micah's care for two years. Confused and unable to rationalize such a huge difference of opinion, I looked up the word 'expert' in the dictionary: *"Very skillful; having much training and knowledge in some special field. A person who is very skillful or highly trained and informed in some special field."* So if what Dr. Bustoff at the insurance company said was true, if he had consulted experts in the field of bone marrow transplantation, what would make their opinions more valuable than those of the experts at two of the top transplant facilities in the United States? I rubbed my temples, fought to clear my head. Something was missing. I could feel it, smell it. Core values maybe. In my mind, it still came down to what I'd been taught by my parents about life, about people, about right and wrong. I was an educated woman with plenty of life experience, and though I was as personally involved in this nightmare as I could possibly be, something ate at my sensibility, something beyond my feelings as Micah's mother, back to the level of him being a human being, a person with rights, with a strong conviction of fairness and truth. What would make the opinions of doctors at the insurance company weigh more than the doctors who knew Micah personally, those who had treated him as a patient and had the opportunity to experience his body's reactions to medications, to hospitalization, to the many procedures and 'studies' he had undergone? How could any doctor read a protocol, a patient history perhaps, and make a judgment call with more authority, more finality, than doctors who responded to Micah, face-to-face, who understand his personal strength, his perseverance through the worst of odds, both assets as important as any course of treatment when push comes to shove.

I spoke with our volunteer attorney, sharing the letter and my growing concern that we might be sent to collections by Ketchell Hospital if we did not make a substantial payment on Micah's account. The bills were now coming to the 'estate of Micah Chase'. It was difficult to believe and worse to acknowledge. It made the hospital seem larger than life; the corporation behind Micah's care seemed as great an obstacle as was the corporation behind our insurance provider. Did the billing department at Ketchell Hospital not know that Micah was a fourteen-year-old child? Though close communication between departments at such a large facility was impossible to expect, it still hurt to see his name written in that context. Micah was a patient who died. His bills needed to be paid. The people in the billing department were doing their job. Micah's charts, the ups and downs of his condition, his heart rate, final respiration, and blood pressure checks had been filed away. Converted to dollars and cents. The hazel color of his eyes, his perfect teeth, beautiful smile, his feet, his lungs, his bones, his body, were no more than a hovering presence around columns of data -- lists of supplies used, services rendered, time spent in their facility. His files had been shuffled from one department to the next, stamped *deceased*, with a time and date, a notation that the account had not been settled, not by any means or with any firm promise of payment.

I was twenty-nine years old when I gave birth to Micah, but my age was not representative of my goals in life. I went to college, majored in geology, minored in anthropology, loved school, would have appreciated a career in either of those fields, but what I wanted most was to have a child -- to be a mother. When I felt Micah move inside my womb for the first time, that flutter like butterfly wings beating ever so softly I knew I was experiencing something I would never forget. The miracle of birth, the primal connection that courses through a mother's veins after birthing a baby transcends death, reaches out with loving hands, nurturing, protecting beyond that mysterious threshold, breaking the most basic of unspoken laws. *You're not supposed to outlive your children. It's not natural. It's not normal.*

That first Christmas was especially difficult. How do you celebrate? How do you decorate? How do you buy gifts for one instead of two? As we had every year, our family met at my mother's house. Grandma Nellie handled Micah's absence with loving grace, placing his stocking in a special place on the window seat in the living room, surrounded by flowers and some toy cars he loved to play with as a small boy. I sat next to the stocking, the flowers, the toy cars, and closed my eyes, recalling another first, one I'd experienced alone months before. It happened just after Micah died and before Del returned home from Texas. Nick was asleep, and the house was quiet. It wasn't quite dawn. My eyes were closed, but I wasn't sleeping. I remember being aware that my mother was there in the living room, on the couch. I knew that people would be coming later in the day to help, to offer support. My mind was working, but my body lay still. The sensation started in my womb, tiny sparks, electric, dazzlingly brilliant, a source of energy so real, so full that it grew to consume me, quieting my mind to everything but it. In waves, one after the other, each stronger than the next, I was filled with a great joy, a peaceful bliss unlike anything I had experienced before. *What's happening?* I asked myself, feeling a little scared. *What's happening?* I asked again. It felt as if a million tiny wings, butterfly wings, were fluttering inside my womb. Like life. Like birth? Micah. The name came out of the depths of my body. I felt him. I knew he was there, that I was birthing him again in a whole new way -- not in a physical body that I could touch and hold, but a spiritual body that I could keep with me forever. *Stay, oh stay,* I begged when I felt him lift above me. *Oh no, not yet! Stay!* I begged again. The sensation was there, and then it was gone, but with it came the feeling that Micah was on his way somewhere else, that he was safe, that he had made it home to me and was off again, flying with his eagles, his angels, on the next leg of his journey.

On December 25th 1993, I sat by Micah's stocking, and Nick sat on my lap. We snuggled, and I kissed him, thinking that tomorrow would be better, that tomorrow I might feel like breathing, like putting one foot in front of the other and getting through a day without tears. I felt blessed to be the mother of two such amazing sons and fortunate to have my youngest still with me. Nick had a way of bringing a smile to my face, no matter what the circumstances. "It's my job to make you laugh," he told me once. A truer statement had never been spoken.

Chapter 18

On January 18th 1994, we celebrated Micah's birthday by taking flowers to the cemetery. We brought a bouquet of balloons, a can of Pepsi Cola, and a Snickers candy bar -- some of Micah's favorites. Someone else had been there -- one of Micah's friends, I thought, or his cousins, Levi and Season. There was a dime and a nickel on a flat stone beside his headstone: 15 cents for my fifteen-year-old son. A fresh smudge stick made of cedar lay half burned in a rusted bowl. There was a single long stem red rose lying crossways on his grave and a Gotcha skateboard sticker leaning against the water urn. Nick put water in the urn, and I put in the flowers we had brought. Del had recently finished building a short rock wall around the gravesite, and it looked beautiful. We had our name, Chase, etched into the stone. I had planted rosemary and some lavender, two perennials I hoped the deer would leave alone. I had also planted two lilac bushes, a Colorado blue spruce and a crepe myrtle, none of which had faired so well. The cemetery was in a rural area and was frequently visited by a family of deer: a large buck, several doe, and a couple of fawns. I had seen a raccoon there early one morning and had heard foxes on occasion barking out a warning to some predator too close to their den. There were squirrels, finches, robins, and dove.

I had seen hawks fly overhead, and I thought, one time, a golden eagle. Micah's gravesite was a peaceful place, and I went there often to think, to cry, and to talk to him.

Two days after Micah's birthday, I received a letter from John Garamendi, the Insurance Commissioner of the State of California. He offered his sympathies and acknowledged how difficult it must have been to experience problems obtaining treatment for Micah while dealing with his illness. Unfortunately, he offered no assurances that the same situation would not happen to another family. *"Experimental treatments are universally excluded from coverage by all health insurers and by all public and private health plans,"* he said, *"and this exclusion is likely to continue in any kind of health care reform."*

Could that possibly be true? If so, it made me angry and frustrated for future patients and their families destined to follow our footsteps. An old saying came to mind: "Never judge a man until you have walked a mile in his shoes." Not for the first time, I wondered what would happen if Dr. Bustoff's son or daughter contracted leukemia or some other life threatening disease. Would he fight for that child's rights? Would he grant payment for their doctor prescribed medical treatment or would he tell that child's doctor to send him home, stating, "This kid is going to die anyway. Why should we put that kind of money out?"

"There will always be some situations in which not all potential patients can be treated," John Garamendi stated in his letter. *"However, in far too many instances, insurers have been arbitrary about what treatments they term "experimental" in order to avoid coverage."*

Mr. Garamendi thanked me for my continued advocacy

on the issue of health care and said he regretted that he could not be more optimistic for a broad change. *"Your letter does reinforce for me the need to address this problem and to continue to seek solutions,"* he added, thoughtfully.

Sometime that same month, I read a newspaper article about a lawyer in Los Angeles who fought and won a case for his sister against the insurance company that denied payment of a bone marrow transplant her doctors had recommended as her best course of treatment. His sister had passed away, as had Micah. According to the article, *Newsweek* magazine had called the verdict "a wake-up call for Washington policymakers." *The New York Times* concluded that "nervous tremors" were being felt in insurance boardrooms across the United States.

My heart pounded as I dialed 4-1-1, requesting this lawyer's phone number, praying that I might finally get some advice that could lead to a resolution for Micah and for my family. I still owed them, my mother, my uncle, my aunt, and friends, $108,000.00. None of them had asked when they might be paid back. Since the day the initial good faith payment was sent to Ketchell Hospital, no one had ever mentioned monies owed or debt unpaid. My family's patience, their thoughtfulness filled me with gratitude, but still, the debt was a stress hanging over my head. Owing my mother and the others for as long as we had, was wearing emotionally on both Del and me. I sometimes woke in the middle of the night and put pen to paper, calculating, trying to figure out how I could send money to the hospital, pay the plumber to fix the leaky pipe in the bathroom and still buy Nick the pair of shoes he needed for school, buy food for the table even. In the dark,

213

alone with my worry, it was hellish. Tears streamed down my cheeks, at times so much so I could not see. Goose bumps rose on my skin as my finger plunked away on the calculator, projecting possibilities, borrowing from one credit card to pay another. The stress was my own; it belonged to me by way of guilt, guilt for what I should have done differently, how Micah's life might have run a different course if only, if only...

The L.A. attorney spoke with me and advised me that based on the information I provided him, in order to win a cause of action, if that was the way I decided to go, I would need to prove there had been a wrongful denial, that the denial had some cause in Micah's death. He suggested I write the highest known person of authority at our insurance company, tell him the background of Micah's hospitalization and request that he again, reconsider.

Following his advice, I wrote Dr. Allison, head of the Insurance Company Review Center, restating the same information I had supplied so often before. The request went nowhere. Again, I received a denial. My friends, Diane Duda and Jan Lekas wrote letters to California senators and assembly members, and I spoke with different attorneys, realizing that our 'pro bono' lawyer, as kind as he was, was a dead end as far as resolution. I became more desperate in the organization of Micah's information. In between helping Nick with his homework, I did my own, making phone calls, speaking with other mothers, people who had suffered the same types of atrocities as Micah. In my sleep, in the shower in the morning, at work, my mind stayed busy trying to sprout ideas through rocky ground. My thoughts had once been fertile with dreams of family and home, but the seeds of new ideas now seemed more difficult to propagate. I tried not to let Nick know that I was as distressed as I was, but he was a smart young man and could tell by the look in my eye when I was with him emotionally or if something was bothering me more than usual. At those times, he was gentle and fun loving, looking for hidden messages from Micah that would make us both smile -- telling a joke, sharing a funny story, simply being himself.

I wrote a letter, mother-to-mother, to former First Lady, Barbara Bush, knowing she too had lost a child to leukemia, and since she was a Texas resident, might have some insight or be able to offer some advice. Though I didn't hear back from her personally, I was told by people at Ketchell Hospital that my letter to Mrs. Bush had been forwarded to the 'appropriate people' with a request for help. Soon I received a letter from Dr. Collier, Associate Professor of Pediatrics at Ketchell Hospital, saying the he had written to the Review Center as well.

March 8, 1994

Insurance Company Review Center
Regarding: Micah Chase

I discussed the protocol on which Micah Chase was treated with Dr. Bustoff of the insurance company in July 1993. It was apparent that a decision regarding reimbursement had been made about the transplant before our brief conversation and that this would be on the basis that the insurance company considered haploidentical bone marrow transplant to be an experimental procedure.

215

I stated that Micah would be the first pediatric patient treated on this protocol at Ketchell Hospital. Four adults had been treated at that time. Dr. Bustoff was told that contrary to his assumption these patients had not died from the procedure and that three had been discharged from the hospital at the time of our conversation. I had earlier discussed the results with our Study Coordinator, in order to give the then most current results when contacted by the insurer.

Given Micah's clinical status at the time and the unavailability of a matched marrow donor, I felt, and still feel, that this was the most appropriate course of action with any possibility of controlling his leukemia.

Sincerely,
Dr. Collier
Associate Professor of Pediatrics
Ketchell Hospital , Houston, Texas

Copies of letters begin arriving in our mailbox, back and forth contention between the insurance company representatives and the newly assigned legal consultant for Ketchell Hospital. New bills and requests for immediate payment to the doctors in Houston, forwarded by their General Council, were added to my growing pile of unpaid bills. I took note of when they arrived and where in the stack they belonged as far as priority. The words 'General Council' merited a place near the top, but in my mind, 'General Council' meant my family was nearer rock bottom. The 'estate of Micah Chase' must have held some accountability in their minds as all letters from Texas were coming addressed this way now.

My father had taught me to buy only what I could afford and to pay my bills as the bills arrived. That philosophy had worked well until the last two years. With my life in a state of lux, the thought of disappointing him was not something I wanted to add into the mix. He had taught me well and been an inspiration for so many things: my love of the mountains, the ocean, sunsets, my children. Along with my mother, he had put my sisters and me first, guiding us through youth, nudging us a bit harder through adolescence and into adulthood. As I thought about my father and the principles of good living he taught me, the principles behind Micah's plight presented themselves yet again. I talked to myself as my father would have talked to me, expressing the truth as simple facts. *Micah wanted his bone marrow transplant. He wanted to live. His fight is an issue of rights.*

No one, especially an insurance company unfamiliar with his person should have had the authority to subjugate those desires, to go over the heads of his doctors, Micah himself, Del and I as his parents, and make the decision to deny treatment. And for a hospital to put the business of money over the business of saving lives, to demand a huge upfront payment before treating a patient in a situation where *weeks* could have made the difference between life and death, was a concept that continued to eat away at my sensibilities. It was no easier to understand now than it was then how this could have happened. I read the most recent letters and reread them, as I had Micah's stories, wanting to understand, to connect with some criteria that made the actions of the health care system we had trusted so out-of-sync with what should have been the case.

The letter from newly assigned General Council, Mary

Wells, was a bill, the first we had received reflecting charges from the doctors in Houston: *"An outstanding balance of $44,150.77 remains unpaid on the physicians account for services rendered to the deceased. If a will has been filed, please furnish me with the probate court, case number. Your response within fifteen (15) days in order that we may proceed accordingly with this case would be appreciated."*

I had issues with this letter, beyond the mention of a will and probate court. Why now, six months after Micah's transplant, were we receiving a bill from his doctors? This was the first of its kind, and their waiting this long confused me. Mary Wells had given me fifteen days to respond. I tagged the letter with a pink sticky note, marked it with a star, and set it aside.

The name on the return address of the next envelope was Fred Jones, Consultant to Ketchell Hospital. Inside were two letters; both were copies of previously sent correspondence. The first was addressed to the Review Center, Insurance Company Managed Care Services, and was from Fred Jones: *"Please be advised that I have been retained by Ketchell Hospital to protect its interest in connection with the estate of Micah Chase. We find your denial of payment of the claims because of "experimental-investigational procedures" being used, to be totally unacceptable. Please consider this letter as our formal request for an appeal of your denial of payment for these services. Enclosed is a letter from Dr. Collier, totally contradicting the experimental-investigational theory that you presented."*

The second letter in the envelope, dated just two days after the first, was from our insurance company. As I read it, I considered the difference in tone from the letters I had received from our insurance company personally: *"By your letter, Ketchell Hospital is appealing the denial by the insurance company for certain services rendered to Micah by Ketchell Hospital. We are, of course, prepared to reevaluate our position, but would appreciate your clarification on a number of points. At this time, there does appear to be substantial evidence to support the insurance company's characterization of Micah's treatment as investigational, including the uniqueness of the protocol under which he was treated, and the apparent lack of prior pediatric experience with this protocol. We will, however, re-evaluate our position and to so do we would appreciate any additional information you can provide."* Frank Lossen, Director, Health Regulation & Operations.

Outside on the deck, with these letters in my hand, I took a deep breath, and tried to relax. Work and school were over for the day. Nick, Chris, and Caitie Deatsch had eaten a snack of yogurt and apples and were jumping on the trampoline in the yard. The air smelled of lilacs. Each year, for as long as I could remember, I had come to wait expectantly for those first buds to pop -- a birth, it seemed to me, on a grand scale. I filled my lungs with the fragrance of the beautiful purple flower as though I could not get enough, as though I could fill and refill and fill myself again and still it would not be enough. Looking out toward the Dardanelle Cones, I thought of Micah, remembering how much he loved to hike and climb the granite domes in the high country. The memory felt good, and then it felt bad, from one to the other in the matter of a second. Parents are tied to their children with a love that runs thicker than the blood in their veins. Most of the things we do in the course of a day, we do with our children in mind -- from the time they are born, until the time we die -- we die. "It's not the child who's supposed to go first," I whispered in echo of previous thoughts. Every part of me is a part of who he was. He had my eyes, my lips. The color of our hair was the same. We even shared the same cowlick. He inherited my love of animals, my lust for life.

I had met mothers throughout the last months, women who had lost *that part* of themselves and never quite recovered. I felt lucky in that way. I had Nick. I endured because I had to. I smiled because it was expected. I may even have felt happy on occasion, but the illusion always vanished just as quickly as it came because a mother's heart is too tied, too bonded, to live every day happy when a part of her has died. People like me -- mothers and fathers who had lost children, aunts, uncles, grandparents were everywhere. I would run into them at the grocery store, at work, at the movie theatre -- someone knowing I was Micah's mom, wanting to share their own story or that of a loved one -- someone who had been left without insurance coverage at a time least expected, whose treatment had been denied, who did not have insurance at all. One day, while sitting on the bleachers at one of Nick's Little League games, I noticed a woman sitting alone. She was staring at the field but beyond it somehow into a world I could not see. Tears rolled down her cheeks, though she did her best to hide them by using her hand as a blockade, pretending to wipe something from her eye, blinking quickly and often, looking up at the sky in hopes of pooling a tear before it fell. When the crowd of parents on the bench cheered her son's name, she came out of the fog, turned, and stared at me long enough for me to recognize something familiar in her demeanor.

"Hey," I said, scooting over beside her. "Great game," I added, giving her time to collect her thoughts, to blow her nose. "Are you Kyle's mother?" I asked, pointing at the boy running past Nick on third base, heading toward home plate in hope of scoring a run for the opposing team.

She nodded her head and looked down, bit at her lip.

"Hey," I said, putting my hand on her shoulder, "Can I help?" I asked cautiously.

"My daughter," she said, "just had her dialysis treatment. She's home right now, but I had to come here to be with Kyle. I needed to spend some time with Kyle, you know?" she said, hoping I would understand. "I don't know what to do," she continued. "Emma's doctor says she'll need a kidney transplant. I don't have money. I switched jobs, insurance companies just before she was diagnosed. They say it's a preexisting condition. They won't pay," she sobbed openly.

I told her about Micah. I gave her my phone number, told her to call, and that I would give her all the information I had, places she might receive some assistance with Emma's medical bills. We talked about the possibility of a fundraiser when the time came. I told her to keep in touch, to let me know how Emma was doing, and where she stood as far as her medical care. Sitting close, breathing the same air, I understood why she chose to sit on the bleachers with the opposing team. I understood why talking to a stranger at that point seemed easier than talking to the mothers, the parents she knew.

As much as I had tried to keep my grief to myself, I felt at times as if I was wearing it all over my face. People expected more of me and more of Nick. The judgmental

221

stares, the disgruntled glares that came our way, the conversations of people who should have known better, were hard to take. "You need to move on," someone would say. "You need to get past this. You know, Micah's in a better place. It's time to let go." Or, "Is it really fair to Nick that you're obsessing about health care reform, about impossible resolutions for Micah's hospital bills?" All I could do was stare at them in disbelief and try to make it home where I could let go and cry in a place no one could hear me.

Sometimes it was hard not to take people's good intentioned statements to heart. I visited the bookstore in town often, browsing through books that explained how I should grieve, laying out the phases of grief in clear-cut steps, precise, and preconceived. I went to a grief support group after a friend told me she feared my sadness was going to have profound and lasting effects on Nick if I didn't get help, if I didn't find a way "to get the smile back on my face." I began stressing about Micah's eternal wellbeing, having been unable to forget a question I was asked regarding our 'Christianity' after his funeral. I had nightmares sometimes, seeing the smirk on the person's face, the way he bounced his foot as he asked me about my religious preference, thinking of Micah lost in some hinterland, unable to gain access into Heaven because of my choices for his service here on earth. I spoke with a minister. I tried to clear my head. The way we grieved seemed tied to the perceptions of the people around us, whether they thought we were grieving enough or too little. Sometimes we appeared to be coping quite well, while at other times our emotional world, our financial world, our family center seemed to be crumbling in front of everyone within eye shot.

In the evenings, when all was quiet, when Nick was asleep, and I was left to my own thoughts, I revisited everything -- my pregnancy with Micah, his childhood on the mountain. As I dug through his files of paperwork, the letters, the bills, doubt crept through the cracks in my heart. Maybe if I worked hard enough I could have changed the outcome; if I could travel back to Oakland Children's Hospital, I would keep a closer eye on his charts, his daily counts. At Ketchell Hospital in Houston, I would be more firm in my beliefs that he was receiving too much medication instead of not enough. Maybe if I concentrated hard enough, I could change the outcome, maybe and finally, I could fix the boo-boo in his bone marrow; I could mend his broken DNA. I worked, and I cried, and I cried as I worked, until I crawled into bed, until Del came in from his garage at night and crawled into bed as well, turning his back to me, protecting himself from my pain.

From the deck, I could hear Nick laughing and felt glad for his friendship with Chris. They had known each other long enough to act like brothers. Though no one could ever replace Micah, having a friend like Chris was a blessing for Nick. Having cousins like Kip, Katy, Levi and Season was a miracle, the way my sisters and I had raised them, so close, so familiar. I chuckled, remembering a week earlier when I kept Levi and Season overnight so Jan could go to a teacher's conference. In the morning, trying to juggle Nick, Season, and Levi, to get them ready for school and out the door by the time Chris and Caitie arrived proved a challenge. Season and Levi were still dressing as we drove off in the car. At their school in Twain Harte, Levi got out of the car. As I turned around to say goodbye, I saw that he had put on Season's pants by mistake. We all laughed and shuffled clothes until they were in the proper places, enjoying a minute of the comedy we had always known together as a family. It was good, and yet it was difficult; I felt guilty laughing without Micah.

Joy had become an unexpected gift. I accepted it, but hesitantly. My world had taken a major shift in direction. Every emotion had taken on a new meaning, and each day I took baby steps toward trusting their validity. Losing Micah set in motion a chain of events I would never have considered had he been alive. My sincere concern for what I saw as an injustice allowed me to tiptoe through my shyness, my lack of confidence, to speak aloud about something I believed in. For the first time in my marriage, I became assertive with my feelings, made decisions when Del was not available to help make them.

The ongoing stresses between Del and me were growing as fast as the weeds in my untended vegetable garden. The slow disintegration of my marriage seemed imminent, but I had no feeling for what could be done, no strength to do anything had I been able to stop it. Dr. Beach had asked me at the beginning of Micah's treatment about the strength of my marriage. The statistics for divorce were high, she said, among the parents of children who are terminally ill. As I watched Nick bounce on the trampoline, I worried about the future, wondering what would happen to us if I were on my own, supporting him and me on the small salary I made at Belleview School. Transitions were not easy. The changes in our lives over the past few years had been devastating. Thinking of what might happen should Del and I divorce, how Nick and I would survive was a possibility I had to disregard. Del was in his own world, pulling further and further away. Avoidance had become his crutch, his way of grieving. It was a necessary step for him, it seemed -- a struggle he needed to go through, an inevitable effort to find his way on the new ground our family walked.

Rather than cancel prearranged vacation plans when Del announced he wouldn't go, Nick and I went on our own. We wanted to visit all those places that meant so much to him and Micah growing up, like the mission at Carmel, the beach, the tide pools at Monterey. We invited two of his friends to come along, and over Easter break, took our yearly trip to the coast. One night on the boardwalk at Santa Cruz, I watched Nick, Colter, and Tommy make a move toward becoming teenagers as they flirted with an entire girl's volleyball team from Canada, the girl's red coats acting like a beacon in the dark, helping me keep track of the young men who had asked me to grant them a little independence. That one stride forward, after so long of slipping backward, was a benchmark of progress for Nick and for me; seeing him boogie boarding, laughing, and playing, sharing our old adventures and memories with his friends with such pride was magical.

In April, I received another letter from the White House, this time from Ira C. Magaziner, Senior Advisor to the President for Policy Development. He reiterated the Nation's need for health care reform, stating that "*fifty-eight million Americans were without insurance,"* and that *"two million Americans lose their insurance each month."* He discussed how the President's new health care proposal would *"outlaw unfair insurance practices"* and would make it illegal for insurance companies to drop coverage or cut benefits, increase rates because of sickness, use lifetime limits to cut off benefits. He thanked me for my continuing support and for sharing Micah's story.

In Houston, Fred Jones, the Consultant for Ketchell Hospital had entered another phase of his investigation and follow-up with our insurance company.

Director of Health Plan Regulation & Operations, Insurance Company
Re: Micah Chase

I am in receipt of your letter of April 11, 1994. Please be advised that I am a Consultant to Ketchell Hospital in their credit and collection department. I had a conference with Dr. Collier and Dr. Klu, and we discussed the questions raised by your insurance company over the time before Micah's transplant. We will now and again, try to satisfy your concerns.

1. Ketchell Hospital as well as many other transplant centers provide bone marrow transplants for patients having acute leukemia in relapse as well as in remission and have determined that remission is not an absolute requirement for a successful outcome.

2. Haploidentical bone marrow as used for transplant under Ketchell Hospital's protocol has been carried out at other cancer centers without T-cell depletion. Our experience does not support the assertion that non T-cell depleted Haploidentical

226

transplants are uniformly associated with fatal graft-vs-host disease.

3. It is a true statement that Ketchell Hospital's protocol follows the bone marrow transplant with a course of administration of Interleukin-2 in addition to standard immunosuppressive drugs given with the intent to reduce risk.

Ketchell Hospital understands that the policy covering Micah excluded experimental or investigational procedures from coverage and we accept your definition of what experimental or investigational procedures are, except that <u>none</u> of the procedures used at Ketchell Hospital are mainly limited to laboratory or animal research. And I am also enclosing a decision handed down from the United States Court of Appeals, 11th Circuit, on August 10, 1993, which is part of the basis of our non-acceptance of your denial.

1. In Dr. Collier's March 8th letter he did confirm that Micah was the first pediatric patient treated under this protocol. The consensus of opinion of the Bone Marrow Transplant Service was that since this treatment had been successful in adults it would certainly be reasonable to believe it would be more likely to be successful in younger persons who are most often more receptive to treatment. It is documented that children tolerated high dose chemotherapy and radiotherapy and bone marrow transplantation much better than their adult counterpart.

2. It is true that Micah was treated under a particular protocol, which was identified as a "pilot study". This means that the doctors were gathering information during this treatment to help them in future treatments, and to share with other cancer centers pediatric departments, but once again, it is not considered "experimental". And after obtaining the experience of four

227

adults being treated, the doctors considered Micah an appropriate candidate in view of his otherwise incurable condition.

3. A consent form is included in every treatment protocol for which data is collected at Ketchell Hospital. The description as a "clinical research study" does not necessarily imply that the procedure is "experimental" or "investigational", only that the protocol has met Institutional Review Board investigation and approval. IL-2 has been used in different conditions, including bone marrow transplant patients, than the labeled use by FDA and has demonstrated anti-leukemia activities. Furthermore, ninety percent of all medications used on children are also used for off label indications.

4. The use of non-T cell depleted haploidentical bone marrow transplantation with IL-2 follow-up in treatment of acute leukemia in relapse is viewed as having progressed beyond limited use on humans and as having become accepted as potentially effective at Ketchell Hospital. And of course, Ketchell Hospital is providing leadership in this area.

The doctors at Ketchell Hospital felt there was no other viable treatment available for Micah's condition.

I have also enclosed a copy of the article short-course Interkeukein-2, Cyclosporine and Steroids for Prevention of Graft vs Host Disease after Hapliodentical Marrow Transplantation presented and discussed at the Fifth Biennial Sandoz-Keystone Symposium on Bone Marrow Transplantation, Keystone, Colorado.

I hope this will help clarify our position in requesting a reversal of your denial of payment of this claim.

Sincerely,
Fred Jones

Suddenly, in California as well as in Texas, refusal of payment on services we thought were paid, were appearing in the form of new bills. In May, I received a statement from the Blood Bank in Alameda that read: *"Your insurance has paid all they are going to pay. The balance is your responsibility. If you have any questions, please contact us."* This bill for blood products, nearly a year after Micah died, was for an additional $11,537.00. Following this, came a letter of intent to send us to collection for the $44,150.77 we owed the Physicians Referral Service in Houston. The monthly statement from Ketchell Hospital was holding steady at $270,000.00.

By now, countless lawyers had turned down Micah's case, most without much more than an introduction. The possibility of putting our house on the market was coming closer to reality. While visiting with my sister Jan one afternoon, after going through scenario after scenario, trying to brainstorm ideas, she thought of an old high school friend who was now an attorney. His specialty was not insurance law, but she thought maybe he could help. Maybe he had some idea as far as the direction we should take. When I phoned Bruce Ramsey, he was thoughtful and immediately responsive. He informed me, as Jan did, that insurance law was not his field of expertise. He also told me that the statute of limitations was close to running out, within a couple of weeks, as far as my ability to file any kind of legal claim against our insurance company. He suggested filing an emergency cause of action on our behalf with the court, to open a case and buy us some time. That first cause of action for declaratory relief was filed in June, of 1994. The push to find an attorney who was willing to help was no longer a situation of wishful thinking, of a cause worth fighting for; it became a matter of urgent importance, an all out push for survival.

A friend at work gave me the business card of a legal firm in Oakland. "Call them," she said. "I've heard they're good, that they care about their clients' welfare and might possibly take an insurance case." The card read: *Gwilliam, Ivary, Chiosso, Cavalli, & Brewer, Attorneys at Law.*

I made the call that afternoon and spoke with an attorney named Eric Ivary. His voice was calming, his manner concerned, and throughout my desperate attempt to tell Micah's story over the telephone, he listened and responded with the message I had waited to hear. "Let's set up an appointment so we can talk at length. Bring everything you have -- letters, bills, paperwork. If we reach an agreement, if we feel that legal action is in your best interest, we'll start by getting the hospital off your back. All contact with Ketchell Hospital will be through our office from this point on. Sound good?"

Chapter 19

The real estate woman I had talked with affirmed what I already knew. The termite problem would have to be addressed, and then cleared by a pest inspection in order to sell the house. I had a pest control service come out and look at the damage. It was more extensive than we thought and would require replacing some major support structure beneath the house. Along with the termites, the technician found bark beetle larvae. This second infestation made the matter more critical. Their potential for destruction was extreme. He thought they had come in with the lumber we had used when we built the perimeter foundation, direct from a local sawmill, some of it green cut. We had also used mill lumber on the inside of the house, lovely blue pine shiplap, and it would have to be removed along with the rest in order to fix the house properly. This became a matter of contention between Del and me. The least expensive route required tenting and fumigating the house. Del did not favor this treatment plan, but to him it seemed the best bet for a lasting outcome. Because of all we had gone through with Micah, however, I was terrified of bringing toxic substances into the house. By tenting and fumigating, the poison would permeate everything -- our cupboards, the carpet, where we breathed, ate, and slept.

Nick was too important a consideration, and I wasn't willing to take such a chance with his health. The second option was replacing sections of wood beneath the house and treating others. Inside the house, we could remove the shiplap and paint the drywall that we had installed underneath. To me, this seemed a safer route, still providing a hopeful outcome. Both options were expensive, the second more so, but it was a step that had to be taken if the house was to be put on the market. And there was still the issue of the leaky pipe in the bathroom. All would have to be cleared by professionals before the house could be sold. The economics of our family structure were spinning out of control. How could we sell the house if we didn't have the money to get the pest work done, the plumbing fixed? The majority was work we could not do ourselves, as it had to be done by licensed contractors. We had placed every board and beam with our own hands, and we were very proud of that. So having hired workers tear apart and repair our home was difficult to imagine and hard to accept. I pushed away any images of how this would all be accomplished, where we would go, and what we would do if the house ever sold. It would not be a matter of selling a home and having the capital to invest in another. If we sold the house, all of our profit would go to Ketchell Hospital. There would be no replacement house other than a rental. We would be starting from scratch, and I knew my marriage would not withstand the stress involved in such a move.

Just outside our front door, my old vegetable garden beckoned me with renegade zucchini vines, volunteers left over from a spring planting in nearby boxes. The large garden area had been fenced off the summer before Micah died, enclosed for the safety of our animals: goats, chickens, a donkey, Alameda the horse. They had all lived in there at one time or another, sharing space, food, and warmth. Opposite the garden was a large wooden shed I used to store feed sacks, a saddle and blanket, lead ropes, hoof picks, some shovels and rakes. I breathed deeply as I opened the door, enjoying the smells of alfalfa hay and old leather as I pulled a large flake of hay from an open bale, pausing only long enough to shake loose the garble of bailing wire that had caught hold of my foot.

As I walked through the garden gate with an armful of hay, I was greeted by Alameda, nudging, and pushing against my chest with his head, snorting happily as I dropped his hay. My sister gave Alameda to me on loan, and I had been surprised by the comfort he had given me. It was Saturday morning. Nick had spent the night at his friend Colter's house. Del was golfing with a buddy. I closed the garden gate and sat down on a cedar stump beside the open fire pit in our front yard, thinking of the last time I had done that, with Micah, just before we went to Texas. We had sidestepped through our conversation that morning, being cautious of each other's feelings, talking about everything but the upcoming transplant.

"Tell me that story," Micah said, "the one you used to tell us when we were little, about Crazy Horse."

"Crazy Horse?" I asked. "You want to hear that story, now?"

Micah nodded his head and settled into his chair, staring at the fire we had built in the fire pit, burning low, nearly out.

"When Crazy Horse was thirteen years old," I began, "he witnessed the shooting of an old Sioux chief by white soldiers on the Oregon Trail. Seeing the dying warrior struck a deep nerve in the boy, and he left camp, traveling alone with no food, no water, no weapons of any kind for protection."

"So when this happened, Crazy Horse was younger than I am?" Micah softly interrupted.

"Yes," I explained. "When Crazy Horse was thirteen, he went on his first vision quest. In those days, going in search of a vision, some truth told to him in the form of a dream, was the way a boy became a man. The way he discovered things about himself, he might otherwise not have known."

Micah closed his eyes, listening. I smiled, and continued the story. "Crazy Horse ascended a high bluff and chose a spot he thought suitable. He fasted and put sharp stones between his toes and pebbles under his body, so he would not sleep. Through the day and night, he lay, then sat, then walked around on his high vantage point, waiting for an answer to his questions, a vision to guide his future.

"He tried to make up songs to sing, but found no inspiration. His eyes burned from lack of sleep. His tongue was thick from lack of water. Through the second day, he waited once more for a message from the spirits. He persisted through a third day, thinking he might be too young and unworthy for a vision to happen. He got sick and dizzy and tried to return to the spot where he had hobbled his pony, but he could not make it. Weak from fasting, he fell down under a large cottonwood tree beside a lake, and it was then that the dream came.

234

"A man with a plain colored shirt and buckskin leggings rode toward him. Up and out of the lake he came on a bay colored horse. In his hair, he wore a single eagle feather, and behind his ear, a small stone was tied in his long brown hair. He told Crazy Horse, "You must never wear a war bonnet or tie up your pony's tail. Before you go to battle, rub yourself with dirt. If you do this, you will not be hurt by your enemy as they pursue you." As the man spoke, his horse became a war-horse, spotted yellow and floating as if in a mist. They flew directly in the path of flying arrows and lead balls, all of them disappearing before they struck him. There was a storm, with dark rolling clouds and thunder, and the man rode through it. A zigzag of lightning suddenly appeared on his cheek, and on his body were marks that looked like hailstones. Over his head at all times flew a small red-backed hawk.

"Some years later, when he was a young warrior, Crazy Horse called upon the personal power of the dream, painting himself with marks of lightning and hailstones, and he wore his hair in the fashion of a red-backed hawk, which he now knew to be his spirit helper. He'd wear his white spots into battle and scream his taunting cry, riding straight through the midst of his enemy, unafraid. Due to his courage, and an unbeatable power that came from believing in himself and in his dream, Crazy Horse became a great warrior for his people."

Micah opened his eyes. He reached down and picked up a piece of charcoal from beside the fire pit. He drew a lightning bolt on his cheek, handed the charcoal to me, and I did the same. We smiled at each other, and laughed, swearing we would never tell anyone what we had done, ran into the house and washed it off before Nick or Del came home. Raising his shoulders high, Micah recommitted to keeping his fear to himself that afternoon, to running headstrong into his own kind of war.

Separated by our growing differences, Del and I stood together for one more fight, for Micah, for Nick, and for ourselves. On Monday morning, we had an appointment to meet Eric Ivary and his partner Steve Brewer. I hoped I could be brave enough to fight in Micah's honor.

I hoped I could keep my promise to him, to make sure we won the war. Everything was organized to go. I had written a six-page documentation of events, had all the letters, the most current bills, all in order by date sent. Auntie Jan would take Nick to school that morning, and if all went well, Del and I would be home in time to pick him up.

Gwilliam, Ivary, Chiosso, Cavalli & Brewer was located in a large suite of offices beside Lake Merritt in Oakland. We rode up the elevator and were greeted by their secretary. She offered us coffee, and after a few minutes, led us to Eric Ivary's office. He and Steve Brewer met us with handshakes, calming us immediately with their warm smiles. I was invited to tell Micah's story in detail.

When I was finished, they agreed to take Micah's case. Just like that, after a year of constant stress and worry, we were able to put our struggle in the hands of two caring and capable men, eager to help us achieve justice for our son. Leaving those offices that day, I cried for a different reason, with relief, feeling some justification that our battle had not been in vain. On July 11, 1994, nearly one year after Micah died, we received a letter from our newly found attorneys. Before I read the letter, I pushed the business card given to me by the Century 21 real estate agent under a potted plant in my kitchen, feeling a glimmer of hope. I adjusted the plant so just a corner of the card was visible.

According to the letter, Eric Ivary had spoken to Fred Jones regarding our hospital bills, and Mr. Jones had been cooperative in that effort, putting to rest any further threat of collection action regarding Micah's account at Ketchell Hospital. Mr. Ivary asked that I forward any upcoming medical bills to his office, along with all correspondence from creditors, hospitals, doctors, and the insurance company. I traced the letterhead Gwilliam, Ivary, Chiosso, Cavalli & Brewer with my fingertips, making sure it was real. My hands shook as I read the letter a second time, verifying what I could hardly believe was true.

As our attorneys began their work, I felt Micah with me constantly. I looked for him everywhere -- in the clouds, in the lyrics of a song on the radio, along the ditch trail as I walked each afternoon. While working at Belleview School, it was easy to imagine him bounding around a corner, laughing, and joking with his friends. His classmates had purchased a beautiful wooden plaque with his name at the bottom as a memorial and had it hung in the school gym. It was a thoughtful reminder of their love for him and a source of great pride for me. As the school librarian, it was my job to read each day to different classes of children, and I loved sharing books with a message. One week, Terri Dixon brought her first grade class in for story time, and I read *The Table Where Rich People Sit* by Byrd Baylor. The story's beginning reads: *If you could see us sitting here at our old, scratched-up, homemade kitchen table, you'd know that we aren't rich. But my father is trying to tell us we are. Doesn't he notice my worn-out shoes? Or that my little brother has patches on the pants he wears to first grade? And why does he think that old rattletrap truck is parked by our door? "You can't fool me, I say. "We're poor. Would rich people sit at a table like this?"*

The story goes on to explain how the boy's father made the table they eat at every day, and he made it out of lumber somebody else threw away. *But my mother thinks if all the rulers of the world could get together at a friendly wooden table in somebody's kitchen, they would solve their arguments in half the time.* The book is beautiful, with vivid imagery, and an ending worthy of discussion. "What makes a person rich?" I asked Terri Dixon's first graders that day. "What makes you feel rich?" I asked again. "Cookies!" someone yelled. "Lots of toys!" said someone else. "Money!" said a third child.

One of Terri's students was Dyllon Bonella. Dyllon had a brain tumor and was a very special friend of mine. We donated the remainder of Micah's trust fund to him after Micah passed away. Having sat quietly through our whole discussion, Dyllon finally raised his hand. "I know I'm rich," he said, "because whenever I look up in the clouds I see my grandma's face. She's in Heaven now, but I know she watches over me. I feel rich because I have parents who love me and a brother who takes care of me and makes sure I don't get hurt." He looked at me with eyes full of understanding and smiled ever so sweetly. Terri Dixon and I looked at each other, neither of us able to speak, both sobbing softly, tears rolling down our cheeks. The rest of the class was silent, staring at Dyllon. Then one at a time they raised their hands with different answers than before. "I'm rich because I have a home," someone said. "I'm rich when the sun comes through my window in the morning," another child shared.

Micah and Dyllon never met, but I felt as if they had. Dyllon seemed to know when I needed an extra hug in the morning, and he would run to me as soon as he got off the school bus, loving me, touching my face, supporting me with his caring blue eyes, his wonderful, bubbly smile. Sometimes he would come up behind me and grab me around the legs. "Guess who?" he would say, laughing. Sometimes in the library he would lean against my shoulder and whisper in my ear. "I'm sorry about your son," he would say. "I love you," he would tell me, before bounding away.

On September 7, 1994, I received another letter from Eric Ivary, saying that the insurance company had made a motion to compel arbitration. He explained that he and Steve Brewer were reviewing the motion and would be doing research in order to oppose it. Should the court grant the motion, it wouldn't be a bad thing, he assured me: "Arbitration can award damages just as effectively as a court and often with fewer legal obstacles and procedures to go through."

It was hard not to feel worried. I knew nothing of motions and arbitrations. I had never had any dealings with the court system, not even for a traffic ticket. On the way to San Francisco once, I got stopped by a highway patrol officer for going too slow. He gave me a warning and sent me on my way. Micah and Nick got a big kick out of that, and it became a standing joke. "You're the only mom we know," they teased, "who's gotten stopped by the police for driving under the speed limit."

My lack of experience suddenly felt like a hindrance, one I needed to correct. As I had with medical terminology, I searched for definitions to those words I did not know or understand. *Arbitration: The settlement of a dispute by a person or persons chosen to hear both sides and come to a decision.* The word and the process were still intimidating, yet it felt better to put a meaning behind the action.

Eric Ivary and Steve Brewer were busy on our behalf. They contacted the Physicians Referral Service regarding their fifteen-day threat of action against us to collect $44,150.77. As I read a copy of their letter to PRS, I felt hopeful, but embarrassed. *"The family is without any funds to satisfy this obligation. I am hopeful that a full recovery can be made against the insurance carrier. There are, of course, no guarantees. However, on behalf of the family I would be willing to discuss withholding funds from the settlement or verdict, if any, in the case which I am handling, in order to satisfy this obligation, provided that no further collection efforts are made."*

It was still difficult to imagine Del and me in the position of being *"without any funds to fulfill our obligation."* Though it was easier knowing that Micah's case was in the hands of our attorneys, the reality of being dependent on other people to correct our financial situation still jangled a nerve in our collective presence. Day to day, we were fine. We had our jobs and received monthly paychecks. It was the medical bills and the reason behind them that caused a gap in our ability to cope.

The one thing Erik Ivary and Steve Brewer allowed us without even realizing it was the time to grieve Micah without the threat of bills and phone calls from collection agencies blocking the process. Micah's friend Jason helped in that process as well, stopping by the house to see if we needed anything, to say hi, and to talk with Nick. Unknowingly, he kept alive a connection to Micah we all desperately needed. As I watched him playing video games with Nick one evening, I felt overwhelmed by his kindness. Other friends of Micah's stopped by regularly too, to check on us, to stay in touch. Jenny, Mindy, and Aaron. Sarah Shaylyn and Christina. My family and friends were a constant source of strength and support, lending an ear when I needed to talk, giving advice when I asked for it. Jan Lekas, Terrill and Denise Deatsch, Patty Young, Diane Duda, Becky Miller-Cripps -- they were there each time it struck me that Micah was not just down the street playing, that he was not coming home. Ever. Every time the feeling hit, it was as if it had not happened before; the blow was that hard and struck that deep. It sucked the air right out of my lungs, made me dizzy, and nauseous, realizing again, and again, that the shoes in Micah's closet were never going to be worn again. The graduation shirt that he had worn so proudly would gather dust on its hanger. I'd call Denise on the phone. "Let's go for a walk," she would say.

"Is it a good time to talk?" I'd ask, calling over and over again, on those people I could count on the most.

Chapter 20

October 4, 1994
Del and Shelley Chase
Re: Chase v. Insurance Company

This is to let you know that the Court denied the insurance company's motion to arbitrate the case. Although the issue was a close one, the Court agreed with our argument that the insurance company did not follow the rules regarding arbitration closely enough to enforce it in this case.

This means that we will now proceed with this case as we would with any other civil case in Court. We will now begin a process known as discovery. This means that we will be sending out extensive questions which must be answered under oath, and no doubt, the insurance company will want to take both of your depositions. We will keep you posted on our progress.

Very truly yours,
Eric H. Ivary

The process of discovery proved long and difficult. Erik Ivary ordered copies of Micah's medical records, but key pieces of information had somehow come up missing at Ketchell Hospital: phone records, fax records, proof that there was a claim by an admissions coordinator in early June of 1993, that pre-certification had been obtained, and that Micah was, at that time, scheduled for transplant. I dug through files, looking for notes I had made. Dr. Beach did the same, as sure of those early conversations as I was, and of the presumption by everyone involved that an approval by the insurance company was forthcoming. In January of 1995, the insurance company attorneys proposed a meeting to discuss Micah's case. Erik Ivary suggested that Del and I meet with him and Steve Brewer ahead of time, to go over a demand which they would then pose to the insurance company attorneys. "Obviously, they are looking for some kind of a compromise figure," Mr. Ivary said, "and they will never willingly pay what a jury would award if everything went our way."

I knew that I had to be ready. It was important that we find the records missing from Ketchell Hospital, as they would substantiate the horror we went through: thinking Micah was scheduled for transplant, and then finding out he was not; being told he was precertified; being told he was not. Out of my stacks of papers, my boxes of files, from the collective memories of myself, Del, and Micah's doctors, our attorneys had to piece together the evidence that would prove the insurance company was negligent in their responsibility to Micah, that their delays to provide treatment, their eventual denial had had a profound effect on his physical and emotional condition. We had to show that Micah's bone marrow transplant was a valid form of treatment for people with Micah's disease and prognosis, that it should have been scheduled and paid for without protest. Most of these facts were surfacing through letters written by the oncologists at Oakland Children's Hospital,

243

the transplant specialists at Ketchell Hospital and the University of California at San Francisco Medical Center. From my point of view, these accumulated facts would be difficult to ignore.

For the first time, it felt like there was a possibility of winning our case. Del and I agreed that we wanted nothing more than for Micah's bills to be paid; we didn't feel right going for a huge sum of money since the point of the case was the issue, and the issue was for the insurance company to pay for Micah's bone marrow transplant. While our lawyers worked, I continued to search for the missing records. In a letter to Eric and Steve I wrote:

"My memory was jogged by looking up this old phone bill. I never keep this part of the bill, so I'm amazed I have this one. I called Pacific Bell and asked that they send me duplicates for the rest of June and July. Someone from the Ketchell Hospital called me very early in June to preregister Micah. Afterward, she sent me a list of housing available around the hospital. The calls reflected on this bill show that I made reservations at an RV Park for the middle of June. I know I had to call back and change the date, at least once, then cancel completely, due to the denials of payment. The first reservation was made for June 17th, the second for June 21st, and I cancelled on June 29th. At that point, we started looking for alternate housing because my mother's motor home was no longer available. I am also sending you a copy of a bill from UCSF to the insurance company that was paid in full. I have found thirteen of those, confirming why we didn't expect any problem with a payment for bone marrow transplantation. Bills were being paid to do donor searching and testing as well. I hope this helps."

In February, Eric Ivary spoke by telephone to Joshua

Rodden of Seycomb, Brasen, Calford & Gifford, attorneys for our insurance company. He then followed up with a letter to reiterate his point. *"The Chase's are very trusting of me and the recommendations which I might make and that gives me a great sense of responsibility, especially in the context of this case. As I mentioned on the telephone, I would not be willing to undergo a dispute resolution discussion where there is not some recognition on the carrier's side as to the potential exposure on the case. I will simply leave it at that."*

I was beginning to understand what Eric Ivary meant by potential exposure. What had happened to Micah, to us, should never have happened. If the facts were presented in front of a jury, if people knew the things that had been done, the things that were said, they might come forward with a positive verdict. Surely, the media would be involved if that were the case. No one would want such a thing to happen to another family, anytime, anywhere. The resulting publicity would not be positive. Eric's letter continued: *"We may have a different view of what this case is about, but it clearly involves both medical and insurance issues. As long as your side recognizes it has a significant exposure and that the Chases' story is an obviously compelling one, I would be happy to sit down in an informal meeting and talk about the case. I would also suggest that my clients be present and that someone from the company be there to meet them and listen to them face-to-face."*

Meeting with someone from the insurance company, speaking with him or her personally, was something I asked of our attorneys early on. I had wished for so long that I could confront Dr. Bustoff face-to-face and ask how he could have been so thoughtless, how his company's gross earnings could possibly have been more important than the life of a fourteen- year-old child. With the reality of meeting someone from the insurance company likely, I was terrified, not knowing if I could hold myself together enough to say what I had dreamed of saying.

I tried to stay focused on finding the items missing from Micah's records. As I had many times before, I phoned Ketchell Hospital and asked to be connected to the records department. I had talked with them often, and they could never come up with the information I needed regarding those first dates of conversations between Dr. Beach and Ketchell's transplant specialist, Dr. Allan, myself and anyone in the admitting department. As I waited on hold, I had a conversation with Micah, as I often did. "This is it," I told him. "If you have any pull, if you can help me at all, baby, now's the time to do it. I love you," I ended, as always. When someone answered the phone at Ketchell Hospital, it was not in the records department where I had previously been routed.

"Archives," the person said.

"I think I've been sent to the wrong place," I said. "I was trying to get to the records department. I've been trying for weeks to get some information about..." I started to cry. I told the person on the other end of the phone, a stranger I had never spoken to before, about Micah and all that had happened. I heard her fumble. I heard her voice shake as she spoke. "Wait a minute," she said. "Let me check something." It took no more than a couple minutes before she was back on the phone.

"These records have been sealed," she said hesitantly.

"What's that mean?" I asked. "What records?"

"It's all here," she said. "The dates you were looking

for, notations about pre-certification. Your son's records," she said. "I have them in my hand."

She agreed to fax them and wished me good luck. I thanked her, and I thanked Micah. As always, I felt him, a little angel on my shoulder, watching out for his mother, his family from afar. There was no explainable reason why I would have been transferred to Archives that afternoon rather than to the person in records department I usually talked with. My son had a hand in this, of that I was sure.

I began dreaming about the hospital again, about dressing changes and blood draws. I still hadn't cleaned out the cabinet in the kitchen where I stored all of Micah's medications, his Broviac supplies. I still had his calendar tucked away in my desk, with the X he had marked as a reminder of the day he would go for his bone marrow transplant. I spoke with Nick, asking him for his thoughts on what to do with the boxes of gauze, tape, and alcohol swabs, the unused syringes, and bottles of Betadine. "Let's give them to Clay and Pat," he said, "to take to the clinic in Mexico." Clay and Pat, our neighbors across the road, went to Mexico twice a year to help supply medical clinics in impoverished areas. It was a perfect idea and so like Nick to come up with it. Together we boxed up Micah's Broviac supplies and carried them across the road, another big step forward for both of us. More importantly, as we walked away smiling, we both knew it was a decision Micah would have encouraged.

Eric Ivary
Gwilliam, Ivary, Chiosso, Cavalli & Brewer
Re: Chase v. Insurance Company

Dear Eric:

We believe that meeting to discuss a resolution could be productive. While we do not mean to imply that the Insurance Company will bankrupt its corporate coffers to settle, we would approach this discussion in a serious and deserving manner. Judicial resolution of this dispute likely will be time consuming and expensive. Further, the Insurance Company is aware of the emotional impact that the litigation may have on plaintiffs, and it has no desire to force litigation should informal resolution be feasible. To assist in evaluating whether a meeting would be a viable option, you agreed to supply us with a settlement demand. We hope that plaintiffs convey their interest in reaching an amicable resolution through the presentation of a reasonable and realistic settlement figure.

Very truly yours,
Joshua Rodden

A formal meeting between the insurance company lawyers, and ours, was set to take place on June 27, 1995. We were fast approaching the two-year anniversary of Micah's trip to Texas. We got news from Heart of America that week that another donor match had been identified from among the pool of donors recruited at one of Micah's bone marrow donor drives; that made six from Tuolumne County alone. Six people had been identified as perfect matches for patients in hospitals throughout the United States; six people had donated their bone marrow for strangers they had never met, for a man, woman, or child who without their sacrifice, might otherwise have died. So again, we celebrated Micah's life. Nick and I took an afternoon and went to Pinecrest with my sister Jan, cousins Levi and Season. We walked around the lake, picnicked, and swam as we had done so many times with Micah. Nick's smile lit my world that afternoon; the black circles that appeared beneath his eyes after Micah died had lightened, were nearly gone. His laugh was healthy and vibrant. Nick's love for his brother was as strong as ever, and he found ways to keep Micah close: through his smile, by telling stories, living his life, and being himself. Those traits are something he and Micah shared, a legacy Nick would continue for himself and for his brother. Living was the one thing Micah wanted Nick to do most. If Nick was living, thriving, if he was happy, Micah's love would be as powerful in death as it had been in life.

Erik Ivary and Steve Brewer asked to meet with us the day before the meeting of attorneys to talk things over and explain how things would work. They explained that Del and my role at this point would be minimal but very important. "The insurance company is interested in discussing the issues," Eric said. "They don't want this to go to trial, and they're willing to discuss a resolution. The meeting tomorrow will be to lay things on the table so to speak." He looked me in the eye before continuing. "You have to understand," he said, "the statements they make are going to be difficult for you to hear."

Erik Ivary shared pieces of some phone conversations he'd had with Joshua Rodden, lawyer for the insurance company, informing us ahead of time what might be said.

"No hospital in California was willing to attempt a BMT on Micah," Mr. Rodden told Eric.

That's a lie, I wanted to scream. *The docs at San Francisco desperately wanted to offer Micah a transplant, would have given him a T-cell depleted transplant if that's what we decided was best for Micah.*

Joshua Rodden states: "The fact is that the research protocol which Micah was subjected to in Houston was so unsuccessful that it was stopped after only five bone marrow transplants. We believe that this experimental protocol was stopped for exactly that reason."

What about the four people who had gone through transplant and were released!

Joshua Rodden states: "It should not be thought that this BMT was somehow covered because it was the only treatment available. It was not. Palliative treatment was available. Micah would have lived longer, in the comfort of familiar surroundings, under those circumstances rather than an early and excruciating death in an unfamiliar hospital thousands of miles from home!"

Going home was not an option for Micah and all of his doctors knew it. Dr. Beach knew her patient well enough to know he never would have settled for that!

Joshua Rodden states: "In our opinion, this procedure was not medically necessary."

Yes it was, damn you, yes it was!

During this first meeting, Del and I said nothing. We listened to our attorneys present our case. We heard the opposing arguments and reeled at the statements being made. At the end of the meeting, a settlement was offered. Our lawyers thanked them but excused themselves and us, signaling the end of any formal negotiations at that time.

During that past year, our case had remained open and pending in the Court of Appeals.

That process was ongoing, as new evidence was presented, as the attorneys and the judges involved in our case debated motions for arbitration. In January of 1996, the Court scheduled an oral argument, at which time both sides were going to ask for a postponement, hoping to pursue a resolution settlement out of court.

A second meeting between attorneys was scheduled for February 23rd. At that time, Del and I would be able to speak personally to the attorneys and a representative from the insurance company.

Cradled in my arms were file folders filled with Micah's medical records, statements from his doctors, affidavits from specialists, letters from the insurance company stating their reasons for denial of treatment -- a pile of hospital bills, two inches thick -- page after page listing procedures, medications given, supplies, from gauze to perc lines. My head swam with medical facts and moral issues, each trying to out-lap the other. "You ready?" Del asked. I nodded my head, but my body said otherwise.

A receptionist greeted us and showed us into a conference room lined with bookcases, hardbound volumes filled with legal procedures and case precedents. She told us to have a seat at a long cherry wood table, offered us coffee or water. Del and I looked at each other but didn't speak, both of us overwhelmed at the prospect of meeting with representatives of the insurance company that had denied our son's bone marrow transplant.

Eric Ivary and Steve Brewer came in to the room first, looking professional but approachable in dark blue suits, light colored shirts, and ties. They greeted us with smiles, handshakes, words of encouragement. Next to arrive were the attorneys representing our insurance company, three of them, dressed in black. No smiles, no handshakes. No greeting. With them was a representative from the insurance company. She was also dressed in black. They took seats opposite us, across the table. Joshua Rodden, attorney for the insurance company, had been waging war for months, reiterating his client's claims: *The doctors in Houston thought of Micah as nothing more than a statistic to add to their research. The insurance company is not responsible for the death of your son. You, and the doctors whose advice you followed, are the ones who should be held accountable.* As I watched Mr. Rodden open his briefcase, shuffle papers, avoiding eye contact, I wondered what kind of man he was, how he could sleep at night considering the nature of his work. I bit my lip and lowered my eyes, hating everything he represented.

Erik Ivary and Steve Brewer had the facts, they knew Micah's story, were prepared to explain the details of his condition and talk about his impassioned desire to live. They were ready to address the insurance company's failure to pay for the potentially life-saving procedure, a medical necessity according to Micah's doctors.

First though, it was up to me. I had prepared a written statement. Wiping away tears with one hand, holding Micah's picture up with the other, I read:

"This is Micah Chase. His was not just a name on a claim form to be dismissed by your clients with the stroke of a pen. He was my child, my first-born son. He was fourteen years old. You can say all

252

you want, make inappropriate accusations, but the fact is you're wrong.

Morally, ethically, as human beings, how could anyone have refused Micah his chance to live? The company you work for didn't know him, how strong he was or how brave. They had no right to assume what was best for him, to play God when it came to his life. The decision to proceed with this transplant was made by his doctors, by Micah, and by Del and me, his parents.

What the insurance company put him through, as far as wasted time, emotional and physical duress, was cruel and unconscionable. As a parent, I am outraged. As a mother, I am lost.

"It's so amazing to me. You think you can put the pieces of Micah's life together. You spout facts as if you were there, with Micah, with us, but the true fact is that you weren't there. I was. We were."

I turned to Del, and put my hand on his shoulder.

"We were with Micah every day. We know what happened. We lived through the events that you've so grossly misrepresented. From a distance, as stranger to him, and to his case, it's easy for you to say that the transplant we chose for Micah was a bad one, but the reality was, Mr. Rodden, that at the time, and under the circumstances, the transplant in Houston was Micah's only option. From the beginning, Micah was involved in his care and treatment. That's the kind of kid he was; he would no more have left his life to chance than he would have given it up without a fight. Don't misunderstand me, we didn't leave the decision about the transplant entirely in Micah's hands, but we knew our child and we respected him as a person. As his parents, we listened and his doctors did the same, recognizing his strength and courage, his love of life, his conviction to make the final choice when it came to his body, his mind.

"The transplant in Houston was Micah's chance to live, and when it came to making a choice, without any hesitation, he chose the

possibility of life over the surety of death, had he just gone home and accepted 'palliative care' as you suggest.

"Mr. Rodden, can you honestly stand there and tell me, that as a parent, if your child faced a terminal disease as Micah did, you wouldn't try everything, do anything, give up your life, your savings, your world, to save his life? To have the chance, Mr. Rodden, to watch your child grow up, to experience alongside him, all that he was meant to accomplish in the normal span of a lifetime -- wouldn't that be worth even a long shot like Houston?

I know what Micah went through in those weeks, while we waited to get an approval from our insurance company. He was smart and observant. He knew what was going on, without us having to explain the details. I know the confusion he felt, the frustration, as he struggled to understand how his life could come down to a matter of dollars and cents. When we were first scheduled to go to Houston in early June of 1993, Micah was strong, emotionally and physically. No one can say for sure if he would have made it through the transplant at that time, but I know my son, and I know in my heart and soul that he would have at least had a better chance. He had the mind set for going through transplant at that time, and no one could have told him any different. "I'm going to make it, Mom," he told me. "Finally, I'm going to get cured." During those weeks of waiting, facing the denials by our insurance company, I watched Micah's spirit fade, his strength weaken. I saw the hell he went through, waiting, wondering. I saw him turn into a shell of the boy I'd raised, and stood helplessly by, as he grew depressed almost beyond hope.

"Micah's physical condition deteriorated immensely during those six weeks of waiting. To you, six weeks may not seem like much, but to Micah, they were everything. By the time we left for Houston, he had gone from a vibrant, happy child, ready for his chance at life, to an extremely depressed child who no longer cared about getting out of bed,

254

who rarely wanted to talk. All he wanted to do was sleep and have me rub his back. His chances for making it through the ordeal he faced were emotionally and physically almost nil at that point. For that, I will always blame the insurance company; regardless of whether the transplant proved right or wrong for Micah, as far as I am concerned, they took away his right to choose. They took his chance for life, and stamped it with a denial.

"Mr. Rodden, no one but God, should have that kind of authority. Dr. Bustoff, with his comments to Dr. Beach, 'This child is going to die anyway. Why should we put that kind of money out?' was out of line and caused irreparable emotional damage to my family. He had no right to play God, Mr. Rodden. No right to sign my son's life away with the stroke of his pen.'"

Chapter 21

In June of 1996, three years after Micah's death, the stress of our debt became unmanageable. After extensive deliberations between attorneys, we accepted an offer and in the insurance company's words, settled our grievance with them amicably. They never admitted guilt, and we never received a verbal apology for the agony Micah went through, or the horror we experienced as a family. But according to our attorneys, the fact that the insurance company agreed to pay the benefits due without a trial was evidence enough that it recognized its liability.

Del and I were required to sign a statement swearing that we would never discuss or divulge any part of the negotiation process. We were issued a check to cover all hospital, doctor bills, and the monies we had borrowed from family. As I held the paper token in my hand, I felt the weight of it measured against the loss of my son. Tears streamed down my cheeks, and I had the impulse to tear the check in half. Why now, and not then, when we needed it most? How could the medical system and the insurance company have failed so miserably when it came to matters of life and death? I threw my head back and wailed a loud, long, guttural sound, just as I did in the hospital on the day Micah died.

Even with the relief of our financial burden, our distress remained palpable. Nick maneuvered through his interrupted adolescence, but he missed his brother terribly and kept Micah's keepsakes close at hand -- CDs and Nintendo games, baseball cards, football cleats and baseball gloves (though he refused to play baseball after Micah died). As time passed, he worked his world like he always did, trying to unite us together as a family with acts of kindness, laughter and play. We struggled to regain some sort of balance, resuming activities we had done before -- camping trips, hiking, sports, and sleep overs, but nothing was the same; the space Micah had occupied was notably empty, and nothing we did could change that. Del withdrew further, and I grew more anxious, focusing my attention on home repairs and activities with Nick. As with any type of verbal abuse, the unjust accusations made by our insurance company continued to haunt me. Their hurtful phrases turned sideways and upside down in my dreams, and in the dark hours of night it was hard not to let those words mutate into self-blame, to think about all the things I might have done differently, before and during Micah's illness.

For solace, I returned to his journal postings: *"I imagine being a doctor someday and treating people for free,"* he wrote just before his transplant in Texas. *"My patients can pay me by bringing me pizza, mint chip ice cream, or changing the spark plugs in my car."*

Del and I had raised Micah and Nick with open hearts; we taught them to look at things positively and dream big, yet all around us, our dreams were falling apart. The added stresses in our lives became too much for us to bear. One weekend, Del said the words I'd been dreading. "I want a divorce."

Distraught and panicked, all I could think of to say was, "Okay."

My mind travels back, sometimes, to those long, hard days in Houston, remembering Micah's tired little body, how hard he fought up until the end. I recall how it was early on at Oakland Children's Hospital, when I had to place my son's life in the care of strangers. As a mother, I watched someone wake my sleeping child to take his temperature, his blood pressure, minister an IV bag filled with platelets, and I felt helpless. The responsibilities I owned as a parent now belonged to someone else. I prayed for caregivers who were gentle, who would appreciate my child for who he is, *was*, before all the craziness started, the illness, the hospitalization, the intrusion on my family's privacy, the constant fear. At Ketchell Hospital, a nurse once told Micah he was "being difficult". She grabbed his arm roughly and moved it to his side. "There, that's better, now stay!" she said, as if he were her pet dog. The experience made me angry, but thankful for doctors and nurses who were not like that: Dr. George, Dr. Feusner, Barbara Beach, and Debbie Atensio, who had been involved in Micah's care for so long.

I now realize that somewhere along the line, in my own search for answers and a hero who might change the course of events, I had overlooked the obvious. The heroes of the world are those like Micah, Maurice, and Dyllon. The heroes of this world are the caregivers of special needs children, and the siblings like Nick who quietly persevere, sacrificing significant parts of their childhood for brothers and sisters requiring hospital care. The heroes of this world are the doctors and nurses who treat sick children with kindness and respect, who fight the corporate giants of the insurance industry for the rights of their patients and the treatments they prescribe.

The boy I mourn is never far away; his sweet smell lingers on his Bugs Bunny shirt and   baseball cap -- his baby blanket, so worn with love that the edging of white ribbon is nearly gone. He lives in my eyes, in his brother Nick, his cousins Kip, Katy, Levi, and Season, in all his friends, and through the lives of people he touched during the course of his short life.

I still cry in the shower sometimes. There are days when my heart lies so heavy in my chest that I can barely breathe. My memories of Micah are good ones, however, and they grow each day, as tiny gifts are added to his list of accomplishments, through Nick and the rest. I visit Monterey and Carmel each summer, and at the Carmel Mission I place my hand on the adobe wall inside the chapel in the same place Micah laid his hand while on our visits there. I light a candle and say a prayer, feeling him beside me, a sensation like a million tiny butterfly wings swirling through my body, his energy as powerful and dynamic as always.

A large bald eagle feather given to me at Micah's funeral sits on a corner stand in a vase in my living room. The porcelain angel Micah and Nick got me for my birthday one year is there too. In a box of keepsakes, along with finger painted pictures, crayon etchings and homemade cards, are Micah's journals. He loved to write. His playful musings are treasured, and the thoughtful reflections of his more

259

serious work inspire me to persevere. I often read the story he wrote at Oakland Children's Hospital before we left for Texas.

Micah's eagles and his angels -- eagle feathers and angel wings -- two very different symbols of two very different ways of thinking have bound together as one in my heart. It makes me smile now, thinking of his precociousness, his courage. *Eagle feathers and angel wings* -- blending ideologies to create something better, stronger.

Imagine what could come of that, Micah. *Just imagine...*

"...One time, with my family in Yosemite, I saw a bald eagle. I've always loved eagles. I like the way they glide in the sky and how they watch over the land. They remind me of angels because of that. I think about eagle feathers being sacred to the Native Americans and angel wings being sacred to people who are Christian.

"I have a lot of time to think right now, and I wonder why people think they are so different from each other. I am in this hospital with kids who may look different than me but we are all really the same. None of us can help where we were born or who our parents are. Here in the hospital we're all just kids. Eagles fly with the angels here. I wish that was true everywhere..."

Afterword

"I remember my brother as the strongest person in the world. He was my hero, and my best friend. Not a day goes by that I don't remember his words and his smile.

I was twelve years old when Micah passed away, and the story as I knew it then, was a Disney version of reality. I appreciate my parents for sheltering me from the medical details and the intense pain my fourteen-year-old brother endured. I am thirty-one now and have a more realistic view of things. I understand what really happened. My wish is that people will read Micah's story, find hope, and gain the strength they need to keep fighting their battles, no matter the reason behind them.

I had the honor of knowing my brother, a fourteen-year-old boy named Micah who died of cancer. He loved life and would have given *anything* for a shot at living it."

--Nick Chase

"Eagle Feathers and Angel Wings: Micah's Story is much more than a story of loss. It is a story about living. It is the story of a family's love that reaches beyond death and gives a glimpse at the miracle of survival in its rawest form, proving that Micah's life was a life worth sharing.

I met Micah Chase in 1991, and was privileged to be his doctor for two years. Micah was an intelligent fourteen-year-old boy, aware of his medical condition, yet full of hope. He was diligent about the care of his body and mind, and had an unshakable commitment to stay strong. Micah would never have surrendered willingly his rights as a patient and human being. To have those rights taken from him by an insurance company doctor, someone distant and unfamiliar with his person and his care, was immoral and unacceptable.

Eagle Feathers and Angel Wings: Micah's Story is timeless and well told. Countless people continue to suffer the same situation as his, enduring the additional stress of unpaid medical bills as they face illness, hospitalization, separation, fear of the unknown. Insurance company denial and up-front payment requirements by hospitals and care facilities occur on a daily basis. As citizens we read about these injustices in our newspapers; as physicians we experience them firsthand. Children suffer, parents agonize, yet the issues of a broken health care system remain unresolved. Money should never be a factor in the quality of health care a person receives. No one should ever profit from another person's misfortune or poor health. All medical care should be nonprofit."

--Dr. Barbara Beach M.D.
Pediatric Oncologist, Oakland Children's Hospital
Co-founder and Medical Director of George Mark
Children's House
www.georgemark.org

"Reading this account, my heart breaks all over again for Micah and his family. I hope they take some comfort from the thousands of donors who were inspired by Micah to join the National Marrow Donor Program and who continue to help other patients now and long into the future."

--Fran McDermott
Heart of America
National Marrow Donor Program

"I am pleased to have the opportunity to offer my comments on Shelley Muniz' touching remembrance of her son Micah. *Eagle Feathers and Angel Wings: Micah's Story* is timeless. Even though these events occurred several years ago, the same problem is happening to other families right now. The story describes the human impact of insurance company greed and callousness on a little boy and his family. The book should help shatter the myth of trust and dependence on the companies which are responsible to pay our medical bills when we need the help.

In the current political climate, much is being discussed about extending health care coverage to every person in our country but little is mentioned about the impact of having health care coverage with benefits that can be withheld because some insurance company decides it can substitute its judgment for the patient's doctors' decision.

Eagle Feathers and Angel Wings: Micah's Story is an inspiring, uplifting remembrance of a courageous little boy and his family and the failure of their insurance company to treat them fairly when they needed the help the most. It will make you laugh, cry and more than a little bit angry. In the end it's a cautionary tale, relevant to the current political discussion, and unfortunately a story that will be repeated again and again until real change in insurance coverage is made.

I highly recommend *Eagle Feathers and Angel Wings: Micah's Story.*"

--Steven Brewer, Attorney
Gwilliam, Ivary, Chiosso, Cavalli & Brewer

Memories

Grandma Nellie Zukal:
"I remember the day I first held Micah in my arms. He was my first grandchild, a beautiful baby, all cuddly and warm. I loved spending time with him and watching him grow. When he was two years old, his grandpa and I started taking him and his cousin Kippy on trips in our motor home. Micah loved our adventures. He loved to hike, and play, and be outdoors. He was a happy boy with a never-ending smile."

Auntie Jan Zukal:
"My special memory of Micah is his love for his family. I remember the laughter, the singing, dancing, learning, playing, loving adventures of life that were theirs to share. Micah touched all of our hearts, but none like the heart of his family."

Auntie Carol Dali:
"My sister Shelley and I found out we were pregnant, each with our first child, just weeks apart. It was very special, being pregnant together, sharing information and learning all we could about how our babies were developing, the newest in birthing techniques, natural childbirth, etc. We couldn't wait to be Moms together. When Micah was born I remember being in awe at how perfect he was. When I would hold Micah, it was as if he knew his cousin was inside of me, waiting to be born. He would become so calm, curling around my pregnant belly,

266

and I would know that the two cousins could hear each other's hearts beating. I truly believe an extraordinary bond was formed during those seven weeks prior to my giving birth to my own son, Kip. Two boy cousins, the oldest of six, became the leaders, giving guidance to the others, sometimes instigating innocent mischief, but always being protective and aware of their role as teachers. Two boy cousins, learning to walk together, starting school together and growing up together. Although Micah's journey on Earth was cut short, his spirit, his laugh, his strength and his courage remain a part of us, always."

Katy Dali:

"The memory that stands out the most for me is Micah's unique laugh that could light up the room. It was not an ordinary laugh, but sort of a chuckle that was contagious. Unfortunately I was eleven years old when he passed away. Shortly after, I remember sitting in his family's living room and hearing my Uncle Del laugh. To my astonishment, it was the same laugh. I closed my eyes and pretended it was Micah in the room with us."

Season Zukal:

"The thing I remember most about Micah was how proud I was that he was my cousin. I loved visiting Belleview Elementary School and bragging to everyone that I was Micah and Nicky's little cousin. Micah was, no doubt about it, the coolest kid I had ever met, and I felt cool just knowing him."

Levi Zukal:

"Micah was like the older brother I never had. He could climb trees higher, jump his bike further, and always had the coolest toys. Nick and I spent countless summer days trying to keep up with him. I'll never forget those times."

Kip Dali:

"Micah and I were born seven weeks apart. We were pretty inseparable. Going up to Sonora, to visit Micah and Nick on Big Hill, was always so cool; there were forts, tree houses, a fire pole to slide on, rope swings -- there was always so much stuff going on, and it was so different than the stuff we did in Modesto. We loved to go to this place called the Uppity. It was a great swimming hole in a creek near where they lived. We'd slide on little waterfalls and look for pollywogs. It was great. One time, my dad was driving an old Jeep on this back road to Micah and Nick's house; the road was really bumpy, and it was storming, snowing. We didn't know if we'd make it or not. Micah opened the window and leaned his head out, patting the side of the Jeep, yelling "Come on, 'ol Betsy! You can do it! Come on 'ol Betsy!" We all laughed so hard. Micah was carefree, always laughing. He was so silly. It was great fun just to be around him."

Acknowledgements

I would like to give special thanks to Dr. Barbara Beach for her dedication to children. She humanizes medicine, and I will be forever grateful for her understanding and light in a very dark time of my life. Thank you also to Dr. James Feusner, Dr. Kelly George, Debbie Atensio, and Nurse Tom for their thoughtful, dedicated care of my son. Thank you to attorneys Eric Ivary and Steven Brewer for believing in Micah and the ramifications of his story.

To all my friends: bless you. To my family, my foundation: my mother Nell, Aunt Nina and Uncle Dave, my sisters, Jan and Carol, my nieces and nephews, Kip, Katy, Levi, and Season, and most especially my son Nick for their constant and unwavering support. And then there is our growing family whose laughter and smiles bring love into my life and foster grand and continuing adventures: Brittany, Courtney, Clint, Kaycie, Evan, Bradley, Kaitlyn, Nathan, Sophia, Gavin, Haylie, Layla, and Landen.

With profound gratitude to: Patricia Kinley, Dr. Paula Clarke, Jan Lekas, Matt Wagner, Michael Knapp, Melissa Colon, and Dimitri Keriotis for believing in the importance of Micah's Story. To my amazing writer friends including Kathe Waterbury, Mic Harper, Arlyn Osborne, and especially my WOW writer's group: Patricia Harrelson, Gillian Herbert, Ellen Stewart, Cynthia Restivo, Suzan Still, Ann St. James, Carol Biederman, and Blanche Abrams. Without their encouragement and a little push here and there, this book would not have been published.

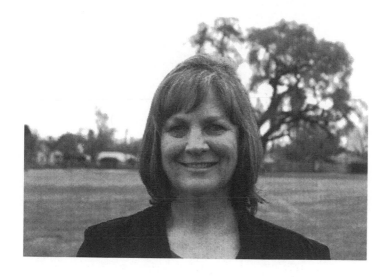

Shelley Muniz lives in the foothills of the Sierra Nevada, near Sonora, CA, and works as a Library Specialist at Columbia College. Her short stories appear in several publications including *Wisdom Has a Voice*, edited by Kate Farrell, *Wild Edges*, and *Wine, Cheese, and Chocolate* published by Manzanita Press. She continues to encourage patient advocacy, the need for health care reform, and supports blood and bone marrow donation.

271

Made in the USA
Charleston, SC
30 August 2013